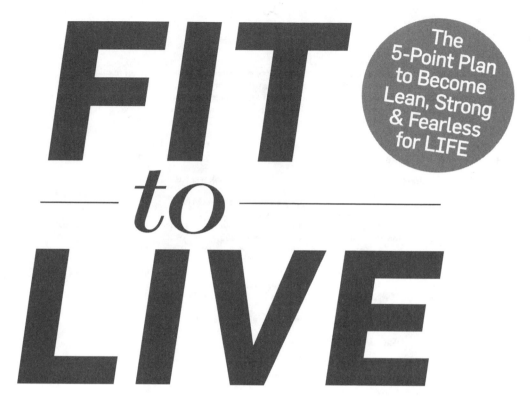

FIT to LIVE

The 5-Point Plan to Become Lean, Strong & Fearless for LIFE

PAMELA PEEKE
MD, MPH, FACP

RODALE

Notice

This book is intended as a reference volume only, not as a medical manual.
The information given here is designed to help you make informed decisions about your health, diet, fitness, and exercise program. It is not intended as a substitute for professional fitness and medical advice. If you suspect that you have a medical problem, we urge you to seek competent medical help. As with all exercise programs, you should seek your doctor's approval before you begin.

Mention of specific companies, organizations, or authorities in this book does not imply endorsement by the publisher, nor does mention of specific companies, organizations, or authorities imply that they endorse this book.

Internet addresses and telephone numbers given in this book were accurate at the time it went to press.

Rodale books may be purchased for business or promotional use or for special sales.
For information, please write to:
Special Markets Department, Rodale Inc., 733 Third Avenue, New York, NY 10017.

Printed in the United States of America

Rodale Inc. makes every effort to use acid-free ♾, recycled paper ♻.

Interior photographs by Mitch Mandel/Rodale Images

Book design by Anthony Serge

Library of Congress Cataloging-in-Publication Data

Peeke, Pamela.
    Fit to live : the 5-point plan to be lean, strong, and fearless for life / Pamela Peeke.
        p.   cm.
    Includes index.
    ISBN-13 978–1–59486–660–9 hardcover
    ISBN-10 1–59486–660–0 hardcover
    1. Physical fitness.   2. Stress management.   3. Weight loss.   4. Nutrition.   5. Conduct of life.   I. Title.
    RA781.P423   2007
    613.7—dc22   2007008698

Distributed to the trade by Holtzbrinck Publishers

2   4   6   8   10   9   7   5   3   1   hardcover

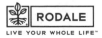

RODALE
LIVE YOUR WHOLE LIFE™

We inspire and enable people to improve their lives and the world around them
For more of our products visit **rodalestore.com** or call 800-848-4735

I dedicate this book to all of you who have taken on life's challenges and have triumphed in the face of adversity. I am in perpetual awe of the extraordinary men and women who have humbled me with their life stories, rich with examples of courage and tenacity. I am blessed to have met so many of you and to have been enlightened by your real-life experiences. I am absolutely convinced that success in the achievement of health begins with a resilient, gratitude-filled, loving attitude toward self and others. From that powerful foundation, the passion for life's journey is born. And from there, meaning for life's chosen paths becomes apparent. I dedicate this book to all of the heroes and heroines who have exemplified this lifestyle.

I think especially of Augie Nieto, one of the greatest figures in the field of health and fitness. As the founder of Life Fitness, he dedicated his life to helping others develop the mental and physical strength to achieve optimal well-being. It is so ironic that the greatest challenge of his life is his struggle with the one disease, Lou Gehrig's, that weakens the very muscles he maintained so well most of his life. Living by the code "in the midst of difficulty lies opportunity," Augie humbly accepted his prognosis and has not let a moment go by when he hasn't kept busy raising millions to fund more research to cure this heinous disease, while loving his family and friends and preparing to leave an extraordinary legacy.

Augie, along with my patients, friends, and colleagues who have embraced adversity with the gusto of the adapt-and-adjust attitude, are my champions in the journey to become Fit to Live.

CONTENTS

FOREWORD

By former Arkansas Governor Mike Huckabee, co-chair of the Clinton Foundation and Alliance for Healthier Generations

L ooking for a really boring snoozer of a health book written by a medical doctor who will make your eyes glaze over with cold technical talk, 20-syllable medical terms, and clinical clichés you've heard a hundred times? Then throw this book away right now, because it is nothing like that. *Fit to Live* will forever change your mind about how you look at weight loss and healthy living.

Presently, many Americans are so out of shape that they can't enjoy a simple family outing because they can't climb a few steps or walk more than a block without huffing and puffing. This isn't just leading to medical diseases, but it's also linked to higher levels of stress, depression, and unhappiness. I ought to know something about being an overweight and under-exercised human. A few years ago, I was obese and a diabetic, and any warnings about a shorter life span went in one ear and out the other. At 5 feet 10 inches and 300 pounds, and only 48 years old, I would pray that after struggling to walk up the stairs at the governor's house, there wasn't a gaggle of reporters waiting to interview me. Why? It would take me 5 minutes to catch my breath, wipe away the sweat from my face, and be ready to talk. I was seriously Unfit to Live. After watching one of my friends, a former governor of Arkansas, suddenly drop dead from a heart attack due to his own obesity and Toxic Belly Fat, I got the memo.

Now, through healthier lifestyle choices, I've removed 110 pounds of body fat, my belly size is well below the 40-inch safety threshold, and I'm no longer diabetic. For that matter, I have the physical exam and laboratory reports of a healthy young man. I find that I'm doing things in my fifties—four marathons—that I couldn't do when I was 18. And I get to do them with my wife, Janet, who's teamed with me to become Fit to Live. I have gone from barely hanging on—being only Fit to Live to survive—to becoming Fit to Live to challenge.

America's health crisis is killing us not only physically but also economically. As a country, we're not Financially Fit to Live. Eighty percent of our health-care costs are due to chronic disease, and most of that is due to three behaviors—overeating, underexercising, and smoking. We spend more of our Gross Domestic Product (GDP) on health care—almost 17 percent—than any other nation on the planet. Most nations spend about 9 percent of their GDP on health-care costs. If we spent 11 percent (still more than anyone), we'd save $700 *billion* a year!

Whether America can remain competitive depends on whether we change our lifestyles to regain our health. There's more cost of employee health care in the cost of a GM car than the cost of steel in that same car! You don't "buy" a car anymore—you buy health benefits for the people who built it, and they are giving you the car for helping them out!

Here's a real call to arms—and legs. We're raising a whole generation of young people who are Unfit to Live and are now beginning to suffer the consequences of their unfit lifestyles. A few years ago, most pediatric hospitals had never seen a case of type 2 diabetes in a preteen. We even called the disease "adult-onset," and type 1 diabetes was known as "juvenile" diabetes. Today, those same pediatric hospitals regularly see cases every week of kids as young as 7 or 8 diagnosed with type 2 diabetes—a disease that once happened to overweight and unfit people in their sixties—not when they were 7! A child diagnosed with type 2 diabetes as a preteen will have vision problems in his twenties, will have a heart attack by the time he's 30, will have renal failure and be on full kidney dialysis by 40, and will never live to see a 50th birthday. Because of the unfit state of America's kids, a child born today is a part of the first generation since the founding of our nation who are not expected to live as long as their parents. This has to change, and it has to start **now,** and it has to start with you and me! The first step is learning how to be Fit to Live long and well.

Dr. Peeke takes on this national nightmare in her characteristically straightforward, head-on, "grab you by the hair and get your attention" kind of way. The result is a whole new way of looking at your waistline and your lifestyle. She'll help you make the Toxic Fat–Unfit to Live connection. Books that make you *think* are good books. Books that make you act are great books, and *Fit to Live* is a great book. Use this book as a step-by-step guide on what to do to get off the couch, get your head out of the fridge, and start living like you plan to stay around for a while. You'll be glad that you decided to get "Fit to Live"!

CHAPTER 1

Are You
Fit to Live?

"It is not the strongest of the species who survives,
Nor the most intelligent that survives.
It is the one that is the most adaptable to change."
—CHARLES DARWIN

I'm here to save your life—if you let me.

First, I'd like you to answer a simple question: Are you Fit to Live?

It's a scary question, isn't it?

In years past, this question basically meant, "Do you deserve to live?" The creepy people who asked this question had usually taken it upon themselves to choose what a good and worthy life looks like.

Here's the reality—we all make that choice for ourselves, every day. There's no external judge or executioner standing around taking measure of you and proclaiming you worthy or not. Your sole judge and executioner is you. You make the decision of whether or not you are Fit to Live by how you choose to think, what you put into your mouth, what you do with your body, how you spend your money, and how you exist in the world. You are answering the question, "Am I Fit to Live?" every day, with every choice you make.

For most of us, the answer is no—*and we don't even know it.*

We live in a post-9/11, post-Katrina world. Be honest—do you really have what it takes to survive life in the 21st century? If you had to suddenly leave your comfort zone and run for your life, hoist your body out of a broken elevator, run after a child headed toward a busy street, or grab a tree limb to stop from falling, could you do it? Are you Fit to Live?

As a physician, my guiding mission is to help people save their own lives. I see my patients struggling, defusing their 80-hour workweeks with buckets of fried chicken, and I know they're not alone. There is a better way, an easier way, a way that will allow you not only to survive, but also to enjoy your life and to challenge yourself, to live big and be bold. My goal is to help you achieve the mind and body that will let you be Fit to Live your dreams. With the plan in this book, I want to help you become Fit to Live . . .

To survive: fit through the exit door of an airplane, lift yourself up after falling, race down four flights of stairs, get through a medical emergency, handle a divorce, survive a financial crisis, be a chronic caregiver without self-destructing.

To enjoy life: sit on the floor with your kids or grandchildren, throw them up in the air without throwing out your back, run along the beach with your dog, garden, swing dance, look and feel fantastic and wear the clothes you love, volunteer in the community, take that yoga retreat.

To challenge yourself: write that book, start your first company, go back to college, become a community activist, start a charitable foundation, walk or jog a 5-K despite a chronic medical condition, rock climb, river raft in the Grand Canyon, bike across New England.

Fascinating FAToid
Can You Make It Down the Stairs?

Forget being able to run downstairs in an emergency. Can you even fit in the stairway? Building engineers tell us that the standard stair width is 44 inches, which was created about 100 years ago when people were thinner. People are now finding it difficult to squeeze down the stairs, especially when they're crowded with others, such as during emergencies like 9/11. This may have been a factor in some deaths. **Bottom line:** Being Fit to Live can save your life.

While the plan is simple, the reality of our lives is anything but. This book is a wake-up call to the fact that our lifestyle has rapidly and fundamentally changed and, for so many of us, become dangerously toxic.

> "The strongest principle of growth lies in human choice."
> —*George Eliot*

We've become not only Unfit to Live to survive life once we're forced out of our comfort zone, but we are actually wearing the weight of our Toxic Lifestyle around our bellies.

Forget about your thighs and rear end. The bottom line is the waistline.

For the first time in history, the bellies of the majority of American men and women are carrying around a life-threatening load of Toxic Fat. Our Toxic Belly Fat gets in the way when we try to zip up clothes or squeeze into the airline or theater seat. This fat is obstructing our ability to run for our lives if we needed to; it's driving us toward a host of diseases and disabilities. Toxic Belly Fat, more than anything else, keeps us from being Fit to Live—to be able to survive, enjoy, and challenge ourselves. To be lean, strong, and fearless.

In 2000, I wrote *Fight Fat After Forty,* the first consumer book about Toxic Belly Fat. Now I'm sounding the alarm that our ever-expanding waistlines are dangerous to our collective mental, nutritional, physical, financial, and environmental health.

⇒Our Toxic Lifestyle⇐
It's a Butt-on-Chair Life

> "Things alter for the worse spontaneously,
> if they be not altered for the better designedly."
> **—FRANCIS BACON**

Over the past half-century, we've been asleep at the meal. Our waistlines have ballooned, adapting to a world of computers, cars, Crackberries, Cokes, and Krispy Kremes. We've morphed from fit primitive physical powerhouses to stressed-out, sleep-deprived, soft-drink-guzzling slouch potatoes. Check this out:

○ The average 5-foot 4-inch woman in the 1950s blew up from a 120-pound, 26-inch waist, size-6 body to, in 2006, a 157-pound, 34.5-inch waist, size-14 body.

- An average guy 50 years ago fit into a 32-inch pant; today he's busting out of his 38-inch belt.
- Already one-third of our children are seriously overweight; many kids ages 1 to 6 are too heavy for standard car seats.
- Teen obesity surgery is the new rage; the number of obese teens has tripled over the past 20 years.
- One out of every three children born in 2000 will have type 2 diabetes by the age of 30. They are the first generation who won't live as long as their boomer parents.

Scared yet? And despite the strong connection between excess pounds and all types of disease, overweight and obesity keep rocketing skyward. In the United States, the rate has gone from 58 percent of the population in 2001 to 63 percent in 2005, and type 2 diabetes has risen right along with it—from 7.9 to 8.5 percent. In just 4 years!

We know that a healthy lifestyle is not rocket science. What part of "stop overeating and move more" are we not getting? Thing is, we've stacked the deck against ourselves. We've created a living (no sidewalks, unsafe neighborhoods, few parks, grab-and-go low-quality eating) and working (long car commutes, elevators, desk jobs, vending machines) obstacle course that seems to make it a mission impossible to achieve health and well-being.

None of these developments, or the others you will be reading about throughout the book, set out to make our bellies swell. But without intending it, we're wearing our stress, lack of focus, and time-starved lifestyle in the form of 30, 40, 50, and even 100 extra pounds.

This Toxic Lifestyle has detached us from our own bodies. Psychologists call it disso-ciation. We eat 24/7 and have no idea what real hunger feels like. We don't know how it

Fascinating FATold

Toxic Baby Bellies

American children and teens are growing Toxic Bellies, a dangerous sign, increasing their risk of heart disease and diabetes. The belly fat of children and teenagers has increased by more than 65 percent since the 1990s—paralleling rising obesity rates. A full 10.5 percent of boys and girls had too much abdominal fat in 1999, as measured by waist circumference. **Bottom line:** If you think Toxic Belly Fat is only an adult problem, you're wrong. This is a call to arms and legs to stop this out-of-control girth control right now!

feels to really use our bodies in a physical way. Our multitasking, distracted minds go a mile a minute. We've lost the ability to focus our time, money, or energy on things that really matter to us. We hide in the cocoon of our comfort zones.

> "You will find peace not by trying to escape your problems, but by confronting them courageously.
> —*J. Donald Walters*

Rather than change our lives, we just keep expanding—plus sizes, seat belt extenders, elastic waistlines, bigger chairs and stadium seats, double-wide wheelchairs and, ultimately, double-wide coffins. We put on "hide-it" clothes—dark colors, loose jackets, elastic waists, XXL T-shirts, baggy pants. The average 36-inch umbrella can't cover most people; the hottest seller is now 48 inches. Most older bath towels are 24 inches by 43 inches, which can't cover the average man or woman, but the new best-selling 45- by 102-inch towels do. We're even too big to fit through the airplane emergency exit row door, especially those small commuter hoppers. Planes take more fuel to get places because we're carrying too much fat.

This Toxic Belly Fat costs us more than our health. Our galloping "globesity" is gouging us financially. By the year 2020, if we keep gaining weight at the current rate, one in every five health-care dollars in the United States will be spent on obesity-related issues in adults ages 50 to 69. That's half again as much as we're currently spending. In 2006, the prime minister of England announced that escalating diseases from obesity, alcohol abuse, and smoking are threatening to bankrupt the National Health Service.

We made history when the World Health Organization declared that there are now more overfed than underfed people on this earth.

This is insane. This is too much fat.

Chances are this information is more than just numbers to you. You're probably at least 20 to 30 pounds overweight, your ever-expanding belly is making you crazy with frustration, and you're teetering on the edge of a host of debilitating diseases. But when people ask how you're doing, you say, "Fine."

We're fooling ourselves by thinking we're fine. We're fine until we're stressed. We're fine until one more thing goes wrong. Then, the comfort zone crumbles, and we have little or no reserves to get through.

I had a 42-year-old patient come in recently who was 75 pounds overweight and on a mountain of medications for heart disease and diabetes. Her opening remarks were "I'm fine. I just need to know how to eat a little better. I'm not interested in exercise."

Fascinating FAToid
Is Your Waistline a Gas Guzzler?

We Americans now use a billion more gallons of gas a year to carry around our supersized bodies. That's enough to fuel 1.7 million more cars a year. **Bottom line:** Who knew that our bodies would have such an effect on our environment? Trim the fat and breathe easier.

A week later she fell down at home, lacerating her lower legs, and didn't have the strength to get up. It took her an hour to crawl to safety, infecting her wounds in the process. Her blood sugar shot up, and she ended up in the hospital for 2 weeks. Then she got depressed and dosed herself with her anesthetic of choice—Ben and Jerry's—blowing up her Toxic Belly Fat and sending her blood sugar and cholesterol through the roof and . . . well, you get the picture. Unbeknownst to her, she'd been sitting on the "fine" line between getting by and utter disaster.

Like this woman, we need to wake up and smell reality. Recently, a guy came up to me tugging on his gut and saying, "I want to introduce you to Bob—Belly over Belt." He and I laughed, but he now knows that to save his life, he must say goodbye to Bob—and so must you.

You deserve to be Fit to Live your dreams. To bound through the day with energy to spare. To wear a belt and tuck in your shirt. To pick up anything off the rack and have it look great. To dance, to run, to have sex with the lights on, to do 10 pullups, to climb mountains if you want to. To feel invigorated and empowered instead of defeated and overwhelmed all the time. *To save your own life.*

Do you think I'm being dramatic when I ask if you're Fit to Live? Let me tell you about another patient. When she first came to see me, Miriam was 61 years old, about 30 pounds overweight, with a belly girth of 38 inches and a cholesterol level of 240. She was dealing with the recent death of her husband and her own retirement. She was overeating, not moving enough, and worried over whether she could live on her pension. Her only solace was her garden. But as she explained to me, "Now that I've finally got the time to garden, it's hard to bend over, I don't have the strength to carry the plants, and I can't see the flowers over my belly."

Miriam began to put into place my recommendations in the Fit to Live categories you're going to learn about. Over the next year, she removed that 30 pounds of Toxic Belly Fat, whittled her waist to 33 inches and her cholesterol to 200, and developed muscles in places she didn't know existed.

One spring day, she called my office and insisted on talking to me. "I finally got it!" she cried. "I need to see you right now."

"Well, I'm with another patient," I replied.

"That's okay," she responded. "I'll share it with them too."

Within a few moments, in she came, tracking mud from her garden and looking scuffed up. She was glowing. "I was in my rose garden, pruning away. Suddenly, I ran into the biggest, hairiest spider I've ever laid my eyes on. I leapt back, stabilizing my legs and grabbing on to the branches behind me for support. As I clung on for dear life, I turned my head and saw the nine stone steps I would have fallen down had I not had the strength to hold on. I firmly planted my legs and pulled myself to safety. Now I really get what you've been talking about! I was strong enough to save my own life!"

Because she was Fit to Live, Miriam did save her life in that dramatic moment—or, at the very least, saved herself from some awful injury and prolonged disability. She not only survived, but she looks and feels terrific and is able to really enjoy her life and challenge herself—by growing decorative cabbages outdoors in Eastern winters, for one. But she also saved her life in a less dramatic way, one that's equally important. By reducing her Toxic Belly Fat, she's reducing her risk for heart disease, diabetes, and cancer.

What's so toxic about belly fat anyway? Well, there are actually two kinds of fat that collect around our middles—outer and inner. The dividing wall between the two is the abdominal muscle. The outer fat is the stuff you can pinch. Some of us have lots of this, others virtually none. The inner fat, however, is like no other. We all have and must have

Fascinating FAToid

Weight Weighs Heavier on Women

Being overweight costs US women 1.8 million years of perfect health and men 270,000. Obesity costs women 3.4 million years of perfect health and men 1.94 million. The researchers suggested that much of the gender difference had to do with the social stigma of weight on women. **Bottom line:** Cut that Toxic Belly Fat and gain your life back.

Fascinating FAToid

Fat Country

People carrying 100 or more excess pounds are so prevalent in the United States that if all those folks lived in one state, it would be the 12th most-populated state in the country. **Bottom line:** We need a Fit to Live revolution to reverse these trends.

this fat. Athletes with low body-fat levels have it. We need it to maintain our core body temperature, to buffer our organs from bumping into one another, and to draw on when we need energy reserves.

So it's a good thing. But like so many other good things, we run into problems when we have too much. Big problems. When there's too much of this inner fat, it interferes with the liver's ability to process cholesterol and insulin, which results in the likelihood of:

○ High blood sugar
○ High triglycerides
○ Low HDL ("good" cholesterol)
○ High LDL ("bad" cholesterol)
○ High blood pressure

Taken together, scientists have named this the metabolic syndrome, but you can think of it as the Toxic Belly Fat Syndrome. You have it if you have two or more of these abnormalities combined with a waistline (measured across the belly button) of more than 40 inches in men and 35 inches in women, no matter what you weigh. And your risk increases as you accumulate more of these five factors.

That's one of the reasons you'll be learning that weight is not really the issue—the size of your waist is. That's also why you may have read somewhere that it's better to be a pear—small waist and large hips—than an apple—round in the middle. It's all about avoiding Toxic Belly Fat Syndrome.

Toxic Belly Fat Syndrome nearly triples your risk for heart disease and increases your risk for diabetes, stroke, and a variety of cancers. It's the main reason that new cases of type 2 diabetes have doubled in the past 30 years, and 41 million other Americans have

DO THE TOXIC BELLY FAT CHECK

Do this in addition to measuring your waistline across the belly button with a tape measure. Lie flat on your back. Take your index fingers and touch your pelvic bones. Even if you have a little fluff there, you do have pelvic bones; otherwise your intestines would be on the floor. Contract your abdominal muscle as if you are about to bear down. Feel across from one side to the other. If your abdominal muscle stays flat, if you have any fat in your abdomen, it's outer fat. If, however, your muscle bulges up like a pregnancy, it means Toxic Belly Fat is pushing your abdominal muscle wall up.

"pre-diabetes," meaning they are at risk of developing the disease. Diabetes can cause blindness, kidney failure, heart attacks, stroke, and the need for amputation. It also increases your risk of Alzheimer's disease.

Women with diabetes are also at an increased risk for glaucoma and, as they age, are twice as likely as women without diabetes to be unable to walk ¼ mile, cook their own meals, or climb 10 steps. (Think about that—10 steps!) Even if you don't have diabetes, high blood sugar impairs your ability to recall information and may cause dementia. As for cancer, apple-shaped men are 39 percent more likely to get colon cancer, and apple-shaped women are 48 percent more likely, and it also increases the risk of rectal cancer.

It's estimated that one in four of us are suffering from Toxic Belly Fat Syndrome, and most of us don't know it. Women are more likely than men to have it. Sixty percent of folks who are obese and 40 percent of those who are overweight are sufferers. But because it's inner fat, you can be normal weight and still have it. You can also be overweight and

Fascinating FAToid
The Expense of Fat
Over 80 percent of the diabetes, heart attacks, strokes, top three cancers, fractures from falls, physical disabilities, and overall complaints to primary-care doctors are caused by the choices we make in our everyday living. **Bottom line:** We look like, feel like, and live like every lifestyle choice we make.

not have it. That's why weight is not as important as the size of your waist. And guess what, people? Science has shown that diet alone won't cut that Toxic Belly Fat. An integrated approach is needed. That's what this book is all about.

Whether you have Toxic Belly Fat Syndrome (yet) or not, chances are two out of three that your waist is too big for your own good. A bigger waist is also linked to erectile dysfunction in men and fertility problems in women, asthma, kidney disease, sleeping disorders, arthritis, depression, and migraines, as well as a host of other diseases. Thick waists are creating fatty livers in kids, which can lead to cirrhosis and early death.

Are we getting all this?

There is hope. I know Cutting Toxic Belly Fat is possible because I've helped thousands of men and women do just that so they could become Fit to Live. Some of them will be sharing their stories of success throughout the book to inspire you.

The Fit to Live lifestyle is not a diet fad or fitness craze. We're so beyond all of that. This plan recognizes that Toxic Belly Fat is not just about how much you eat and how little you move. Rather, it's about how and where you live, how much you have (or don't have) in the bank, how you think about the world. This plan "sees" the whole you and helps you get started, no matter where you are. This simple but comprehensive approach puts it all together with the tools you need to look stunning, feel invincible, and live a more fearless, joy-filled life.

⇨Fit to Live⇦
Your Waistline Will Thank You

> "And in the end, it's not the years in your life that count.
> It's the life in your years."
> —ABRAHAM LINCOLN

Cutting the fat and becoming Fit to Live is about creating *reserves*. Specifically, Body Dollar reserves. When we deposit Bank Dollars, our goal is to have what we need to live on day to day and to build reserves so that we can draw upon them in times of future need. We feel secure when we have reserves in our Bank Dollar account. That's good wealth management.

We also have a Body Dollar account. Every time you practice Safe Stress, eat well, and stay active, you're making deposits to your Body Dollar account so that

> "I intend to live forever. So far, so good."
> —*Stephen Wright*

you'll have reserves to draw on. Manage your Body Dollars well, and you'll cut Toxic Belly Fat, which enhances your ability to survive, enjoy, and challenge yourself. It's not a matter of "if" you'll need that reserve to save your life; it's a matter of "when." Being Fit to Live is all about learning how to build your Body Dollar account, use it optimally, and maintain a reserve to help when the going gets rough. That's good health management.

Science tells us that, if we do things right, humans now have the potential to live for 100 years. So this isn't just about getting into a bikini—this is about optimizing the quality and quantity of all the years of your life.

Take a look in the mirror. Is the body you see going to take you to 100? In other words, do you have the Body Dollar reserves you need, both for day-to-day functioning, as well as for any potential emergency? Can you hop out of bed in the morning, energized and able to tackle the day's stresses? Embrace every day with an inner core of empowerment and self-confidence?

Now, I'm not guaranteeing you'll live to 100. Accidents and genetics play important roles as well. And don't think you can rest on your parents' or grandparents' longevity genes. As they say, genetics may load the gun, but environment pulls the trigger. Banking Body Dollar reserves optimizes your environment.

How do you figure out the state of your Body Dollar account? Like a bank statement,

OPEN YOUR BODY DOLLAR BANK ACCOUNT TODAY

Try this practice inspired by my patient Cindy McCrae, who's removed 42 pounds of Toxic Belly Fat. Put a sign on your mirror that says, "How many Body Dollars will I earn today?" Then put one on your fridge that says, "How many Body Dollars do I want to spend today?" It will help you understand it's all about Body Dollars in and out on a daily basis.

Fascinating FAToid

Alert and Vertical Alert!

Want to decrease the chances of ending your life in a nursing home? Smoking in middle age increases the possibility of ending up there by 56 percent, while high blood pressure increases those odds by 36 percent, and lack of exercise by 40 percent. Type 2 diabetes triples your chances, and diabetes plus any of the other factors increases your odds fourfold. **Bottom line:** Put that cigarette down. Get up and take a walk. Now is the time to create the Fit to Live lifestyle.

you need to look at the numbers—belly size, cholesterol, blood sugar, blood pressure, body-fat percentage. Work with your doctor to collect that information and get the all-clear to do something about them. Then you need to consider functional components. Can you get up those stairs, walk that mile, run for your life, adapt and adjust (which I like to call "A^2") easily? The Fit to Live plan will help build a program perfectly suited to your current Body Dollar balance. Knowing you're optimizing these numbers and abilities as best you can leaves you with a wonderful sense of security and satisfaction.

Great, you say, I'm ready. But I'm tired of being battered by conflicting opinions about exotic supplements and complicated exercises and meal plans.

I understand how you feel. Sometimes, I feel overwhelmed by it all—and I'm a doctor whose job it is to pay attention!

Fortunately, it's really not that complicated. I'm a bottom-line person. So here it is: In all my years as a fitness and nutrition expert, a scientist, as well as a practicing physician, I've worked with everyone from inhabitants of Capitol Hill to glitterati in Hollywood—and I have yet to meet anyone who doesn't want to live independently as long as possible and then die in their own bed.

Sister Genevieve Kunkle, one of the famous Notre Dame nuns studied by aging expert David Snowdon, PhD, professor of neurology at the University of Kentucky, is a great example of this Fit to Live attitude. She once noted that the secret to her success at achieving centenarian status was quite simple: "I have two good traits. I am alert and vertical."

Well, in a nutshell, there's your long-term goal. To remain Alert and Vertical so you can look and feel great and live mentally and physically independent—for a lifetime.

Life is really all about choices. I'm going to dare you to look at your future and plan for tomorrow by making wise choices today. You can read this book and do nothing differently—that's a choice. But I am going to make sure you know the consequences of that choice.

Becoming Fit to Live has five elements, what I call the five Ms:

- Mind (Are You Mentally Fit to Live?)
- Mouth (Are You Nutritionally Fit to Live?)
- Muscle (Are You Physically Fit to Live?)
- Money (Are You Financially Fit to Live?)
- Macrocosm (Are You Environmentally Fit to Live?)

I introduced the Mind/Mouth/Muscle template in my book *Body-for-LIFE for Women*. At that point, I'd been using it with my patients for years, and I'd seen it help a great many people. But even then, I sensed something big was missing, something that could actually encompass the entirety of real life.

You've seen by now that when people come to me to talk about removing pounds, they eventually see that their problems don't necessarily begin and end with what they're eating or drinking—or even how they're dealing (or not) with stress. More and more of my patients are starting to bring up money troubles—I'm talking big fear, either of losing it or of not having it to begin with. (Sound familiar?) Others are being driven nearly insane by chronic clutter, disorganization, and toxic living environments. (You too?)

After hearing story after story like this, it became apparent to me that the original template couldn't capture the whole picture. In response, I've added two new Ms—Money and Macrocosm—to my approach, and the results have been tremendous. I've been stunned.

Over the years, I've seen that each of the five elements is crucial in and of itself. Each has consequences—positive ones if we make the Fit to Live choices, negative ones if we consistently choose to remain Unfit to Live. But what's critical to understand is that each element also supports and enhances the others. Check out how this works:

- When you Cut the Belly Fat (Muscle and Mouth), you earn more (Money).
- If you have greater income (Money), you can afford better food (Mouth) and that gym membership (Muscle).

Fascinating FAToid

The Body Dollar Payoff

A study comparing Seventh-Day Adventists to other Californians found that a healthy life-style added 7.3 years to a man's life and 4.5 to a woman's. And they were healthier years, with fewer pills, operations, and hospitalizations. **Bottom line:** Cut the Toxic Lifestyle Fat, and you'll have more energy and look better too!

○ When you are physically active and looking great (Muscle), you feel better emotionally (Mind).

○ When you practice Safe Stress (Mind), you don't stress-eat (Mouth). You have more energy, so you declutter your home and get rid of toxic relationships (Macrocosm), which makes it easier to focus on the other Fit to Live elements.

That's why, when I talk about cutting the fat, I'm not just referring to Body Fat. I'm also talking about Mental Fat, Financial Fat, and Environmental Fat. Becoming Fit to Live is about cutting all our Toxic Lifestyle Fat.

To cut the fat and create those Body Dollar reserves, you're going to have to pay a bit more attention than you probably have until now—to thinking right, moving right, eating right, spending and saving money right, and living right. Sure, you'll spend some Body Dollars, but just like with a savings account, you'll get more back than you put in.

As you begin your Fit to Live journey, you'll immediately notice a surge of energy, better sleep, and an increased sense of self-esteem and achievement.

If you're overweight or obese, you'll pare 3 inches off your waistline within 4 weeks. You'll remove 2 to 3 pounds (women) or 3 to 4 pounds (men) of body fat every week.

> "You are in control of your life. Don't ever forget that. You are what you are because of the conscious and subconscious choices you have made."
>
> —*Barbara Hall*

Within 6 to 8 weeks, you'll drop a full size (or more) as you become stronger and leaner. And you'll continue to refine your body composition until you reach your Fit to Live goal.

You'll feel less depressed and anxious, more hopeful, empowered, and focused. You'll notice that your home and workspaces are less cluttered. You'll manage your short- and long-term finances better, and you'll bank dollars to live healthfully for a lifetime.

It's okay if you haven't been good with self-care till now. That has nothing to do with how smart, successful, or nice you are.

> "Insanity: doing the same thing over and over again and expecting different results."
>
> —*Anonymous*

But becoming Fit to Live takes a new skill set, one that you will be learning throughout this book.

To create your personal Fit to Live plan and start to Cut the Fat, you'll first take the Fit to Live assessment test at the start of each section. These tests will place you at one of three levels: Survive, Enjoy, and Challenge. Once you have your scores, you'll learn what these levels mean for your current health and well-being. Get ready for some pretty startling prognoses for your future.

At the Survive level, your Fit to Live goal is to learn the basics to survive not just your daily living, but to begin to bank some Body Dollar reserves to draw upon during crises in any part of your life. The Enjoy level means you've got Survival nailed, and you can expand further outside your comfort zone and bank more reserves while applying what you now know to enjoy life at a deeper level. The Challenge level means you're already Fit to Live

Voice of Success: Enjoying Her Reserves

Valerie Szabo went from a 37-inch belly and 35 percent body fat to a 29-inch waist and 20 percent body fat and maintained for 5 years

"Being in great physical shape with Dr. Peeke's plan has been a godsend because I am coping with a diagnosis of lung cancer, and those Body Dollar reserves have helped me recover more easily from surgery. I have now had several physical therapy sessions, the huge mass of scar tissue on my side has been reduced drastically, and my pain has subsided significantly so that I am no longer taking any pain medication. I just did a 30-minute cardio workout and two sets of weights. I'm regaining strength and looking good. I'm very excited about what I've been able to do with my Body Dollar reserves."

BECOME FIT TO LIVE
TO ENJOY AND YOU WILL . . .

IN 4 WEEKS

✓ Shed your Toxic Belly Fat, paring 3 inches off your waistline

✓ Remove up to 2 to 3 pounds (women) or up to 3 to 4 pounds (men) of body fat every week

IN 6 TO 8 WEEKS

✓ Drop a full size (or more)

IN 12 WEEKS

✓ Build 3 pounds of muscle

✓ Increase your metabolism by 7 percent

LONG TERM

✓ Save your own life and potentially other people's if faced with a life-threatening event requiring reserves of physical strength and stamina

✓ Add on average 8 to 9 high-quality and joyful years to your life with your positive attitudes and stress resilience

✓ Reduce your waist size to the normal range (women less than 35 inches, men less than 40 inches)

✓ Improve your ability to use glucose fuel in your blood by 25 percent and increase bone mass by 1 to 3 percent

✓ Reduce your cholesterol levels

✓ Slow the aging process, maintaining healthier skin, shinier hair, and stronger bones

✓ Enjoy a healthy body composition (weight, fat, muscle) for life

✓ Cut your risk of dying young by 25 percent

to Survive and Enjoy, and you are ready to push beyond your previous limitations, push your envelope, and challenge yourself to achieve your dreams.

You may be at different levels in the five categories. For instance, you may be at the Challenge level in Mind, Enjoy in Money and Macrocosm, and Survival in Muscle and Mouth. The tests are designed to help you figure out exactly where you are so you can design a program that works for your individual needs and goals.

To help you become Fit to Live, Cut your Toxic Belly Fat, and move yourself to the next level in each of the five areas as quickly as possible, I've taken all the science on health and

✓ If your blood sugar is high, you'll cut your risk of developing type 2 diabetes by more than 50 percent

✓ Reduce your risk of heart attack by 65 to 90 percent and also reduce your risk of strokes; colon, prostate, pancreatic, and breast cancers; osteoporosis; and impotence

✓ Reduce arthritis-related joint swelling and pain (if you don't have arthritis, you'll prevent it from happening)

✓ Relieve any menopausal hot flashes and headaches by 50 percent

✓ Relieve symptoms of depression by 50 percent (equivalent to taking antidepressants) and get increased feelings of happiness, well-being, self-esteem, and confidence

✓ Sleep better while preventing and potentially reversing sleep apnea

✓ Reduce the risk of Alzheimer's by up to 60 percent and improve overall brain function, including memory and attention

✓ Delay the onset of disabilities associated with aging by 12 years

✓ Save $2,200 a year on medical bills if you're over 50

✓ Be able to pay for a long and joyful life in an environment that revitalizes and refreshes you

wellness and boiled it down to basics. The "Our Toxic Lifestyle" sections in each chapter will help you understand how we got into this predicament to begin with. Then, we'll move immediately to solutions. I've distilled the screaming headlines into five simple Fit to Live Principles in most chapters. These principles form the basis of my bottom-line advice for each level—the Fit to Live Essentials.

This plan is meant to work with you, wherever you are today. If you're gung ho and want to take yourself on right now, go ahead—you'll achieve results much faster. However, if you want to ease into it, starting with one new strategy per day, that's fine too.

The chart in Appendix 2 will help you track your results based on your preferred level of commitment.

As you progress, go back and retake the tests to watch yourself move through the levels. You may start out just hoping for survival, but trust me—you're headed for a much better place. I'm not exaggerating when I say that once you hit the Fit to Live to Enjoy level, your entire life will start to change. (See "Become Fit to Live to Enjoy and You Will . . ." on page 16.)

The goal is to become someone who can become Fit to Live and manage the five Ms by yourself. But you might need support for a while, and that's what this book is designed to give. In addition, my Web site (www.drpeeke.com) offers a wide range of resources to help you in Mind, Mouth, Muscle, Money, and Macrocosm, as well as individual and group support. Once you take the tests, read each section, and begin to put Fit to Live Essentials into action, you'll know we're there, if and when you need more help or someone to talk to.

I won't be asking you to do anything I don't do. I believe in walking the talk. And as your guide, I'm issuing you a challenge: Starting right now, whatever your age, gender, or shape, shout out loud, "I take myself on!" From now on, you're going to bank your Body Dollars, Cut the Toxic Belly Fat, and celebrate every day you live and breathe.

Are you ready to be Fit to Live?

If not now, *when*?

Let the journey begin.

PART 1

Mind: Are You Mentally Fit to Live?

"The mind possesses and is possessed by all the ruins
Of every haunted, hunted generation's celebration."
—DELMORE SCHWARTZ

This section addresses the question, Am I Mentally Fit to Live? To Survive, to Enjoy, to Challenge—and to save my life?

The only way to Cut Toxic Belly Fat is first to Cut Mental Fat. That's why the Fit to Live journey starts with your head. Getting your head screwed on right will power you through tough times and keep you on track.

To be Alert and Vertical as long as you can, you need a powerful reason to become Fit to Live: It's all about creating meaning so that your life becomes a wonderful adventure you want to hop out of bed for. In Chapter 2, you'll learn the science of change—how to create the changes you want in your life and develop the positive attitudes that will sustain those changes. You'll learn my most important strategy: A^2, or adapt and adjust. Then, in Chapter 3, you'll learn how to use A^2 to cope with life's stresses in a way that minimizes Self and Health Destruction and conserves Body Dollars. You'll even learn why A^2ing will save your life by helping you live an additional 8 to 9 years! By the time you finish this section, you'll have a more powerful, fearless voice, one that says I deserve better, and you'll know the simple actions you need to take to remove Mental Fat *for life*.

To begin, find out your current level of Mental Fitness. Choose the answer that most closely matches your situation:

1. When under high stress—such as you owe the IRS more money, your kid's flunking school, your weight's up 25 pounds—your typical response is to:
    a. Become depressed, withdrawn, irritable, and angry, taking it out on others.
    b. Occasionally vent to family and friends, experience some sleepless nights, but you keep trying to regroup.
    c. Rely on your spiritual life, taking time to pray or meditate while adapting and adjusting each day.

2. During a checkup with your doctor, she sees that you're under a lot of stress. Because you have heart disease in your family, she warns that the stress may impact your health. Your response is to:
    a. Blow her off and say you'll get to this sometime when things calm down.
    b. Read her brochure on stress management and occasionally try a few breathing exercises when you're anxious.
    c. Immediately take yourself on, make an appointment with a counselor, buy a meditation CD, and start to practice breathing exercises.

3. For you, as you go through each day, you feel:
    a. Out of control, with everyone else and their needs controlling your life.
    b. Able to get at least 50 percent of your to-do list accomplished.
    c. Satisfied that you have achieved your personal and professional goals for the day.

4. You see your friends:
    a. Frequently. Your schedule is full of plans for dinner, coffee, visiting museums, etc.
    b. Occasionally. You wish you could see them more, but everyone (including you) is so busy. You end up constantly scheduling, canceling, and rescheduling.
    c. Rarely, and you have only two you've stayed in touch with over the past 10 years.

5. If someone asked you to explain the purpose of your life, you'd:
    a. Have no ready answer.

b. Be intrigued by the question, realize you've thought about it occasionally, but don't feel prepared to discuss it without more thought.

c. Be happy to share your personal insights and relate your work, personally and professionally, with your life purpose.

6. Your mother breaks her hip and is hospitalized. You're the primary caregiver. Realistically, this means that:

a. You stop exercising and eating well, begin to worry constantly while you're getting only 4 hours of sleep every night.

b. You're able to get the basics of life done—your job, the grocery shopping, picking the kids up from school—but you're exercising less and occasionally stress-eating.

c. You take healthy food to eat when you stay with her at the hospital, and you bring your sneakers so you can get a brisk walk in through the hospital corridors.

7. Each night, you are typically getting how much sleep?

a. Fewer than 4 hours a night

b. Between 5 and 7 hours

c. Between 7 and 9 hours

8. If you're feeling depressed or anxious, you're most likely to:

a. Have a glass of wine or scoop of ice cream.

b. Neutralize stress with any combination of exercise, meditation, sharing with helpful friends, and journaling.

c. Self-destruct with overeating, drinking, smoking, and/or taking drugs.

9. While walking alone at night, you hear someone coming up behind you quickly, so you:

a. Panic and freak out, drop your belongings, and begin to run away.

b. Try to stay calm and alert as you look around for a place with people and safety.

c. Clutch the pepper spray in your pocket and mentally replay what you learned in self-defense class.

10. Your company has just been sold, and the new personnel manager announces that 40 percent of the staff will be laid off. You:

a. Divide your time between bitching with co-workers and sending out résumés.

b. Seize the challenge and immediately put the word out to your contacts, send résumés, and avoid the water cooler rumor mill and gossip sessions.

c. Start smoking again.

Scoring:

For each Mind question, match your answer to the proper score.

1. a, 0; b, 1; c, 2   6.   a, 0; b, 1; c, 2
2. a, 0; b, 1; c, 2   7.   a, 0; b, 1; c, 2
3. a, 0; b, 1; c, 2   8.   a, 1; b, 2; c, 0
4. a, 2; b, 1; c, 0   9.   a, 0; b, 1; c, 2
5. a, 0; b, 1; c, 2   10. a, 1; b, 2; c, 0

Add up your score and check the key below.

0 to 6: Fit to Survive. You're barely Mentally Fit to Live. You survive day to day by jumping from one crisis to the other, and you're winging it with your self-care. The day-to-day stresses of life keep your mind so cluttered and overwhelmed that you can't imagine actually having time to enjoy your life, much less take on a challenge like losing weight or getting a promotion.

Having higher depression is associated with a 29 percent increased risk of acquiring excess fat in the inner abdomen and Toxic Belly Fat Syndrome (metabolic syndrome) over time. Higher anger scores were associated with a nearly 50 percent increase in risk of the full syndrome—Toxic Belly Fat, heart disease, and diabetes. If left untreated, high levels of anxiety and depression put adults of all ethnicities at a two- to threefold greater risk of developing hypertension serious enough to require medication. Clinical depression is associated with increased risk of heart disease and heart attack for men.

7 to 13: Fit to Enjoy. You're the typical model of the Mentally Fit to Live man or woman. You've been banking some precious Body Dollar reserves by continuing to show enough stress resilience to make it through the day. For the most part, you manage to carve out time to exercise, spend time with your family, and enjoy what matters most. You adapt and adjust to daily stresses, and you hit your mark 70 to 80 percent of the time. Because of this, your chance of avoiding or minimizing the impact of disease is excellent. You're in great shape to live your full life span.

Your strong network of friends and confidants significantly reduces your risk of premature death. Men and women with the strongest network of friends were 22 percent less likely to die in a given time period than those with the weakest network of good friendships. Friends may exert a healthy influence on risky behaviors, like smoking and drinking, as well as have important effects on mood, self-esteem, and coping with stress.

14 to 20: Fit to Challenge. You are the Mentally Fit to Live super-achiever. You feel in control of your life and your destiny. You have a better handle on the meaning of your life and what gives you joy. You embrace adversity and see each stress as another opportunity to challenge your stress resilience skills and to learn. Fit to Challenge men and women are banking the largest amounts of Body Dollars. This super-achiever reserve will shorten healing time when you experience a medical condition, and maximally optimize your life span. Many Mentally Fit to Live to Challenge folks are highly spiritual—and people who attend religious services at least once a week are less likely to die in a given period of time than people who attend services less often.

Bottom-Line Results from Becoming Mentally Fit to Live to Enjoy

■ You'll be able to save your own life—if seriously stressed—with the Body Dollar reserves you've banked.

■ For every pound of Mental Fat you cut, you'll cut 10 pounds of Belly Fat by eliminating self-destructive behaviors.

■ Your Power Why will guide you through any of life stresses and keep you on your healthy lifestyle track.

■ You'll add on average 8 to 9 high-quality and Joyful years to your life with your positive attitude and stress resilience.

■ You'll stay youthful, both mentally and physically, and will be at lower risk for dementia, memory loss, sleep impairment, low sex drive, heart attacks, obesity, and other stress-related health woes.

CHAPTER 2

Cut Mental Fat to Reduce Body Fat

"Life is largely a process of adaptation to the circumstances in which we exist. The secret of health and happiness lies in the successful adjustment to the ever-changing conditions on this globe; the penalties for failure in this great process are disease and unhappiness."
—HANS SELYE

The story goes that tennis legend Billie Jean King was coaching Zina Garrison when the young pro was having some hard times. One day, Billie Jean just looked at her and said, "Champions adjust!"

Amen, sister! And all of us are champions of our own lives—Fit to Live champions. Billie Jean understands what the great stress researcher Hans Selye proclaimed decades ago in his important book *The Stress of Life*—things change, and to succeed, we must too. If you don't know how to adjust, you end up paralyzed, anxious, and carrying around tons of mental weight that ends up as Toxic Belly Fat.

Through my years of research and work with patients, I discovered the key to weight control. *Cut Mental Fat to reduce Belly Fat*. That means not only having a mind capable of change, but also knowing how to get out of Mental Fat habits that can otherwise sabotage your efforts to become Fit to Live.

⇒Our Toxic Lifestyle⇐
A Tsunami of Change

"The truth does not change according to our ability to stomach it."
—FLANNERY O'CONNOR

In the past, we didn't have to cope with a lot of change. Of course, people changed to survive when the times called for it. If the hunt wasn't successful, if the crops didn't come in, they adapted by going lean and mean until they had more food resources. Wars and depressions happened, and folks tightened their belts and made do. However, for most of human history, the pace of change was, in general, slow. If you were a gardener for the king of England in the 17th century, you were a gardener your whole life, and so was your son. Your grandson too. Human beings tended to stay in one place for generations and lived much shorter lives. The change they had to deal with was basically just births, deaths, and marriages.

With the advent of technology in the 20th century, however, change is now hitting us at blinding speeds. Twenty years ago, I was typing my research on a typewriter. Remember those? What about VCRs? Do you even remember the last time you used one of those?

Nowhere are these rapid changes more evident than in the number of jobs we hold. Compare the number of lifetime jobs 45- to 65-year-olds will have—two—to the number of jobs 15- to 45-year-olds will have—*eight*.

Fascinating FAToid
No Wrinkle Issues

For 99 percent of human history, the average life expectancy was less than 18 years. During the Civil War era, the average life expectancy was 30 and the most frequently cited cause of death was "exhaustion." By the year 2050, scientists estimate there will be 1 million centenarians. **Bottom line:** If we're to live to be 100, then our goal is to live long and live well. That's what becoming Fit to Live is all about.

Fascinating FAToid

Paying to Be Thinner?

People surveyed said they would be willing to take off 10 pounds and keep it off if paid $225.

Bottom line: I don't believe it. They'll drop the weight and gain it right back. This is short-term change for a quick buck. The only way to Cut Belly Fat for life is to Cut the Mental Fat.

Along with techno creep and career bloat have come tremendous changes in how we live. We don't have to go out and kill ourselves scoring a meal. There's cheap food to be had on every city block. We don't have to make our clothes or build a home. We just buy it all. No calories burned, yet lots of food passing through our lips.

In response, everyone is looking for the magic formula. We don't take time to learn *how* to change, to get into action and stay focused. As a result, people keep repeatedly losing and finding the same Toxic Belly Fat. How about you? Ninety percent of us make New Year's resolutions (the top one being lose weight), and only 8 percent succeed.

Instead of seeing it as a reality to be accepted, we spend a great deal of time pushing

Voice of Success: Waking from the Food Coma

Terry Garland removed 130 pounds of Toxic Body Fat and has kept it off for 12 years

"Firmly implanted on my beat-up couch, I used to watch the world go by. I went to work, came home, grabbed food, and plopped onto the couch, feasting until I was satisfactorily anesthetized from the pain of my existence. One day at age 40, the only guy in my life dumped me. Being dumped by a loser made me race to the fridge. But I had no appetite. Just a strange surge of energy as I began to awaken from my usual food coma. I was angry. The pain of living the way I was finally exceeded the pain to change. I decided to reverse everything I'd been doing. I gave the couch away, started walking, blew off junk food, volunteered in the community, made new friends, and got a new job. Today, I work in the health-care field, helping others change their lifestyles."

> ## BOTTOM-FEEDING MENTAL HABITS
>
> Take a look at these self- and health-destructive mental habits. Have a favorite?
>
> **Bitch, Moan, and Whine (BMW):** Why me? It's not *fair*. I shouldn't have to go through this.
>
> **The Mental Cuisinart:** I can't believe she said that about me. Why would she do that? Am I a bad person? Why hasn't she called?
>
> **Total Stress-Out:** Oh my god . . . not another change! How am I going to cope with this on top of everything else? I can't deal with this. I can't handle one more thing!
>
> **Going Postal:** How *dare* they do this to me? No one treats *me* this way. I'll show them.
>
> **The Scarlett O'Hara:** I'm going to ignore this. If I just pretend it isn't happening, maybe it will go away. Any day now, things are going to go back to the way they were.

against change or denying that it is a permanent fact of life. When change comes at us, rather than putting our energy toward finding the best solution possible, we tend to go to the Dark Place and Bottom Feed. You know, that's when you get caught in festering, self-destructive ruminating like a catfish sucking up all the nasty gunk at the bottom of a pond. You Bottom Feed when you pout, blow your top, stuff your face, or dissociate.

Women are hardwired to spend vast quantities of time in the Dark Place, ruminating on what to do, how to do it, why we haven't yet done it, and why it's so unfair that we have to. Men Bottom Feed with aggressive, chest-pounding tactics or abject silence and withdrawal.

We all have our own special ways of health-destructing. You might socially withdraw from people: "Naw, I don't want to go to that party." Or you put a negative thought in your Mental Cuisinart, hit chop and high, and let it spin for hours. Or you overeat, smoke, overdrink, do drugs, or spend like you're as rich as Oprah. Any of those things deplete your Body Dollar reserves and interfere with your ability to be Fit to Live.

It's time to get out of the Dark Place and stop Bottom Feeding.

⇒Fit to Live⇐
Optimal Thinking from Now On

"We would rather be ruined than changed;
We would rather die in our dread
Than climb the cross of the moment
And let our illusions die."
—W. H. AUDEN

Those who remain Mentally Fit to Live for as long as possible understand how to adapt and adjust (A^2) with a minimum of health-destruction. Whether the change is expected (an upcoming wedding) or unexpected (an illness), they A^2 so they can achieve.

Imagine your boss walks in the door and says that your job is being eliminated due to restructuring. You could get drunk, eat yourself into a food coma, shoot the guy (only kidding!), trash the company to everyone you know inside and out, cry for months, or go into a funk and lie on the couch until your unemployment insurance runs out. This is Bottom-Feeding behavior—knee-jerk reactions rather than conscious responses.

Bottom Feeding is expensive. You'll spend a lot of Body Dollars. Plus, these habits do nothing about getting you what you really need, which is another job.

The A^2 response goes like this:

Adapt: Adapt is a mental attitude that says, "I'm facing a situation that I have to come to terms with." You're a human being; you'll have a wave of emotions about the situation. But the better you know how to adapt, the sooner the wave can dissipate. It's about accepting the situation—I'm going to lose my job—with as minimal negative effects on yourself—shame, guilt, anger, denial, inertia, stress-eating—as possible. Once you do that, it's time to . . .

Adjust: Adjust is about asking yourself, "Given this new reality, what actions do I need to take to get the best results possible under the circumstances?" It's about formulating a plan, a strategy to respond to the situation in a healthy way. In the

> "Vision without action is merely a dream. Action without vision just passes the time. Vision with action can change the world."
> —*Joel Barker*

case of a job loss, that might be to get great recommendations, see your company's benefits office, put the word out about what you're looking for to everyone you know, and so on.

The trick is to A^2 as quickly as possible so you don't spend a lot of time in unhealthy responses that you have to recover from later—gaining 30 pounds or racking up $1,000 on your credit card. You'll know how to A^2 when you truly get it that change needs to be embraced as a natural part of life. The more you adapt and adjust to that one fact, the less time you'll spend fooling yourself that any day now, things will calm down and stop changing.

Why do we fear and resist change so much? Brain science estimates that 90 percent of our daily lives are lived in habit—we get up and shower and brush our teeth the same way each day, eat the same breakfast, drive the same route, eat the same lunch, come home and watch the same shows on TV, over and over. Habit conserves energy—we don't have to think about things we do habitually.

But habit is bad for the same reason—we're on autopilot. Remember that last birthday party you went to? How did those two servings of cake get in your mouth? The same way they did the past 30 times you did it.

When we want to change something in ourselves, habit is not our friend: "Oops, I forgot to order salad instead of pizza." "Oops, I forgot I was going to the gym after work."

We can break this cycle and change a habit by making a different choice. The more you practice the healthier choice—say, exercising instead of drinking—the stronger the new

Voice of Success: The Tree Ate My Treadmill

Deborah Kinney removed 50 pounds and has kept it off for 5 years

"My husband and I were going great guns with weight removal. Then one day, there was a big thunderstorm. A gigantic oak tree crashed into my bedroom, destroying not only the room but also my treadmill. In the past, I would have gone into an eating frenzy to numb the pain of having to rebuild. Instead, I remembered what I've learned about adapting and adjusting. I looked at my husband and said, 'Honey, I've been meaning to redo the house, and the bedroom looked like heck anyway. Now, we'll have some money to be able to redo it.' I'd always been fragile when it comes to change, so I took a chill for a couple weeks to regroup. Then I picked myself up and went back at it."

habit becomes. Eventually, you don't have to work so hard to remember to choose it.

The challenge here is that the old sequence is lurking in the part of the brain concerned with habits and addiction, waiting to re-emerge if something kindles it. That's why, under stress, we often return to things we stopped doing years before. The good news is, once you've created the healthy choice, you can return to it much more easily because you already have a strong pathway in your brain for the good option.

Admittedly, the mental work of change really causes your gray matter to sweat big time. I remember when I first discovered that while an undergraduate at the University of California at Berkeley. I was taking an organic chemistry course with Melvin Calvin, the famous Nobel laureate. One day, a very brave kid asked a question. Calvin hated to be bothered with questions. Somewhat irritated that the question was a good one, Calvin didn't directly answer but spun around and began writing the answer onto the multiple chalkboards behind him, making it so confusing that the kid actually said, "This is hard!"

Melvin Calvin flipped around, locked eyes with this undergrad, and yelled, "Are you in pain, young man?"

The young man responded, "Yes, this is quite painful."

Then Calvin smiled more broadly and said, "Good! Now I know you're learning!"

I never forgot that learning is painful, and it's supposed to be. That's why I teach each person to expect and embrace the mental sweat it will take to change. As I have helped thousands of men and women get Fit to Live, I've discovered that change actually happens in steps, each of which has its own layer of Mental Fat. As you read, think about what stage you're in.

THE SEVEN FIT TO LIVE STAGES OF CHANGE

1. Obliviousness

Obliviousness is where you're not even aware of the need to change. Perhaps the pounds have crept on slowly. After all, it takes a gain of only 2 pounds a year—the average weight gain during the holidays—to be 20 pounds overweight in a decade.

In this stage, you avoid looking in the mirror. You buy bigger sizes and live in elastic without letting it register consciously. You don't think about the fact that you never exercise. Your blood pressure may be high and/or you're becoming insulin resistant, the sign of type 2 diabetes. Somewhere in the back of your mind, you may know you're not handling the stresses of your life well, but it's not registering on the conscious level. Psychologists call this dissociation the capacity of the mind to dis-connect from the emotional or physical pain we're experiencing. It's a good thing for sur-viving traumas such as war, rape, or car acci-dents. But it gets in our way when we need to allow our pain to touch us so that we can become aware we need to change. People can hang out here for years, even decades.

> "You have to allow a certain amount of time in which you are doing nothing in order to have things occur to you, to let your mind think."
>
> —*Mortimer Adler*

If you have a sneaking suspicion you're dissociated, seek the appropriate help: a social worker, psychologist, or coach. Or start with a trusted friend who's a straight shooter. They may help you finally tell yourself your True Truth, your uncensored, no-holding-back-bottom-line-raw-truth about yourself and your situation.

2. Someday I Will . . .

This stage is when you admit that maybe you have a teeny-weeny problem. You're starting to feel some inner stirrings of discontent. Instead of avoiding the mirror, you take a closer look. But your inner voice says that you'll deal with it later—when your child leaves home, when things settle down at work, when you come back from vacation—any date will work as long as it's *not now*. No rushing into things. If you are here, there are all kinds of "good" reasons your mind cooks up for why it's important not to do anything quite yet. You can hang out here and defer change endlessly.

How will waiting one more day help? It won't. In fact, it will just groove in the bad habits that much more. *If not now, when?* Wake up and smell reality: The sooner you get into positive action, the sooner you will see positive results.

3. The Wake-Up Call

One day, you "get it." The time for change is now. Mostly, people don't come to see me until they reach this point. I'm always curious to find out what did it. They often say some-thing like, "It's time to feel better and get healthy."

I say, "Oh come on. Now tell me *what really happened to get you off first base.*"

And it will be something like: "The scary vacation photos" or "When my doctor put me on meds for high cholesterol and high blood pressure" or "When my husband/wife started to make comments about my appearance and my habits."

My good friend, Arkansas Governor Mike Huckabee, told me that despite a fresh diagnosis of type 2 diabetes, skyrocketing cholesterol, and blood pressure issues, he was not motivated to do anything about the 300 pounds on his 5-foot 10-inch body—until one day, a former Arkansas governor, equally obese and unfit, was getting ready to come to the Huckabees for dinner and dropped dead from a massive heart attack. When he'd learned what happened, Huckabee turned to his wife, Janet, and asked, "Is that me?"

"Yep" was her response.

The next morning, he was at his doctor's office, and 1 year later and 100 pounds lighter, he'd run his first marathon.

For most of us, the wake-up call comes when we allow our pain to touch us. As a resident, I remember seeing a husband and wife in my clinic. I followed them for about a year and then saw the wife a year and a half later. She was 50 pounds heavier. I walked right by her in the waiting room because I didn't recognize her.

It turned out that since I'd last seen them, her husband had been diagnosed with pancreatic cancer and died only 45 days later. "It was the worst time of my life," she confided. "We barely had enough time to get our act together. And after that, I just couldn't cope."

I went to my mentor to discuss the case. She said, "Ah yes. The widow pounds."

Ever since then, I've seen it time and time again. The caregiving pounds. The rotten marriage pounds. The passed-over-for-promotion pounds. And I've encouraged men and women to name those pounds. Because when you do, you make the *pain–pounds connection*. It's your Belly Fat brought on by your Mental Fat of struggling with life's stresses.

I once keynoted a health conference for the women of Microsoft. I said, "Look down at

Fascinating FAToid

It's Never Too Late

Even if you've waited until your golden years to start getting healthy, you will reap benefits. Seventy- to 90-year-olds who started eating right and exercising for 30 minutes daily were half as likely to die as those who didn't during a 12-year research period. Of course, if you start younger, you've got a much better chance of being Alert and Vertical well into your later years. **Bottom line:** Never let your age or a long history of health destruction hold you back from starting your Fit to Live journey today.

your body, and if you have excess weight, think of what precipitated your weight gain and then name those pounds after that stress." During my book signing after, a young woman came over, her eyes misting. "What you said struck home," she said. She was only 31 and very successful. She had moved from Switzerland to Seattle because she'd been given a big promotion. She'd never had a weight problem before. But she missed her old home and family, leaving her chronically depressed and 25 pounds heavier in the course of a year and a half. She looked down at herself and said, "These are Seattle pounds. I want my Switzerland body back.

"You know," she went on to say, "I walked into your talk with a huge candy bar in my hand. After listening to you, I left it on my seat. I called my husband and said, 'We're going back to Switzerland.' There was a dead silence and then he said, 'What took you so long?'"

The wake-up call comes when you become aware that the tried-and-true ways of numbing yourself from the pain of your stress—overeating, alcohol, drugs, anger, withdrawing from friends—are not working anymore. Instead, like this young woman, you begin to notice a visceral feeling of discomfort that cannot be neutralized by your old health-destructive habits.

When the wake-up call comes, there's a Click! in your head. It's when you realize that the pain you'll feel from changing will be far less than the pain of staying where you are.

4. Humble Acceptance of Needed Actions

This step is when you stop fighting this simple truth: To be Fit to Live, you have to do the work in all five elements of your life—Mind, Mouth, Muscle, Money, and Macrocosm. You just have to. Period. Just like you don't fight against taking a shower daily, it makes no sense to fight against the actions you need to be Fit to Live.

I first experienced humble acceptance as a young girl. Like with all kids, my mother said to me, "You've got to brush your teeth every day." She went into a scientific explanation about cavities, which went in one ear and out the other. I didn't want to do it. Every morning and night, I threw a little toothpaste under some water and lied through my teeth (pun intended) that I had brushed ever so thoroughly.

Then I went to the dentist for the first time. He discovered three cavities and came at me with the needle and drill. Suddenly, brushing my teeth wasn't so bad after all. I swore I would do whatever it took to avoid this guy with his pain machines. I had gone to the place of humble acceptance.

Through scientifically based studies of people who are successful in long-term lifestyle changes, we now know that in *every* single instance, there is a humble acceptance point. After the wake-up call click, there's a peaceful place you settle into where you don't spend any more Body Dollars complaining about the work of changing. Instead, you humbly accept what you've got to do from now on.

5. Getting into Gear

Here's where you look at Mind, Mouth, Muscle, Money, and Macrocosm and come up with an action plan based upon small steps that you gradually incorporate into your daily lifestyle. Remember you have to A^2 as you live out the plan each day. When the going gets tough, be prepared to aggressively fight off instincts to go back to the Dark Place and Bottom Feed.

The good news is that I've done the heavy lifting for you by providing the Fit to Live tests and the Fit to Live Essentials in each M. Some of these may be things you're already doing—great! Others, you'll have to decide how to fold into your life. When, where, and how depends on your personal circumstances.

When you create your plan, don't bite off more than you can chew. If you make a grand

Voice of Success: Fit to Live to Love

Sharon Daniels shed 25 pounds in 12 weeks and has kept it off for 1 year

"I'm 28 and have been married for a year to Jeff, a terrific guy. He's a short guy, but he's buffed and takes good care of himself. Since our wedding, I'd put on 25 pounds, and it started to change our relationship. I didn't like myself anymore, felt tired, and started to withdraw from him. My wake-up call was when we were getting intimate one night and I realized that I now weighed more than him and was probably squeezing the air out of him when I lay on top of him. I decided at that moment that I'd had enough. Under Dr. Peeke's guidance, I learned to keep focused on the most important objective—my relationship with Jeff. I did the work and shed the pounds. Only then did I have the self-esteem to try getting physical again. After a wonderful Christmas party, we tumbled into bed and after a joyful reunion, Jeff yelled at the top of his voice, 'I love Dr. Peeke!' When I told her this story, she turned beet red."

Fascinating FAToid

Believe and Live Longer

Those who have faith give themselves a boost to their immune systems and are less likely to experience anxiety or substance abuse. Believers also tend to exercise more, smoke less, and have lower blood pressure and cholesterol, which means a reduced risk of stroke, heart disease, or dying of cancer. **Bottom line:** Having a strong spiritual life can help you make the changes you want in your physical life.

plan to do every suggestion in every chapter, you will most likely not succeed at any of them. I suggest you start by adding one tip a day, and build from there.

6. Staying Focused with Your Power Why

Your Power Why is there to help you when it all boils down to a choice to bank those Body Dollars or not. It must be really simple, or it won't work when the doughnuts are calling your name. You're either going to eat the doughnut that's sitting there or the yogurt and walnuts you brought to work—and your Power Why will help you make that choice. (Develop your own in "Create Your Power Why" on page 37.)

This Power Why is like an invisible 2 by 4 to your head. It wakes you up from your stress trance, keeping you mindful of the consequences of your choice. As you stare at the doughnut, you make the connection. You say your Power Why—your 7-year-old son's name, "Jeremy"—and you remember you want to be healthy and alive to take care of him and see him through graduations and grandchildren. By rejecting the doughnut—junk—and choosing the yogurt, you're choosing Jeremy.

The choice is simple: Jeremy or junk. The choice you make is what you will look like, feel like, and live like. In this way, your Power Why is your friend when you're down and out with exhaustion and stress.

I think of Zoe, a beautiful, smart 13-year-old, who inherited her father's obesity gene. The child of a stressful divorce, she was overweight and unhappy. She'd tried a number of weight-reduction programs, but nothing stuck. When we met, I asked her what gave her joy. What she dreamed of. In a word, it was Broadway. She was a fantastic singer and as she fell asleep each night, she sang and danced on Broadway in her dreams. Her Power Why? Broadway or no way. Every time I see her, Broadway's been winning.

7. A²-ing for the Rest of Your Life

When times get tough and you don't manage stress well, I never say you've "relapsed" or "fallen off the wagon." Every misstep is a golden opportunity to A² and move on.

For instance, let's say I have a business dinner at 8 p.m. Do I want to go? No, it's too late for me to eat. Am I going to sit around and whine? Or resign myself to ordering a big plate of fried chicken and french fries? No. I'll A². I'll eat responsibly all day, get my exercise in, have a yogurt before I go in order to calm my appetite, and eat lightly. Ideally, if they have it, I'll have a salad, a serving of protein, some vegetables, and perhaps a little fruit.

A² means you think ahead and plan to stay on track. That may mean creating Plan A, Plan B, or even Plan Z if you need to, because all kinds of things are going to come up that could get in your way if you let them. Your mother breaks her hip. When you A², rather than giving up exercise for the duration of her hospital stay, you walk up and down the hospital corridors for 30 minutes every day. Going on a long plane flight with nothing served but a variety of high-fat, low-quality carbs? When you know how to A², you pack some nuts and dried fruit.

A² is a vaccination that gives you the ability to stay Alert and Vertical when life hits. The most common reason people cite for bailing on themselves is unexpected change. I hear things like "I was perfectly fine, shedding pounds, and then my husband had an affair." Or "I just found out that my son is flunking college."

How about you? Think back to the last time you were derailed from your healthy lifestyle program. I'll bet you'll say, "I was doing just fine until _____ [fill in the life event] happened." Sure, if a serious stress occurs, your self-care may go straight to the dogs. For

Fascinating FAToid

Those Ugly Days

When women feel bad about themselves, two-thirds of them say it's because of their looks or their weight. **Bottom line:** Stop looking in the mirror for the answer to your angst. Look deeper, and you'll see the root of your anxiety. Face off with the real stresses, A², and make the changes that will truly bring you joy and fulfillment.

a week, 2 weeks, a month. That's understandable! But the better you get at A^2-ing, the shorter the time it will take for you to regroup and move on.

Mentally Fit to Live folks *plan* for problems. When you do have a setback, treat it as temporary so you don't lose much momentum. Take the lesson and incorporate it into your daily A^2 practice.

⇒Fit to Live Essentials⇐

Using your score from the "Are You Mentally Fit to Live?" test, you'll start to build your individual program with the tips below. Begin according to your current level. If you're at the Survive level, focus on the first section, and really master these baseline skills before moving on. If you're at the Enjoy or Challenge levels, feel free to scan the first section(s) to see if there's something you might need a refresher on; otherwise, move to your section, try those tips out, and appreciate what life is like beyond survival mode! To keep yourself on track, check out Appendix 2 for a template that will help you organize your individual plan.

TO SURVIVE:

If you received a score of 0 to 6 on the test, focus your energy here first. Once you've mastered these, feel free to move up to the tips in "To Enjoy."

1. Name Your Mental Fat

What stresses gave you your Toxic Belly Fat? If you can identify them, you can develop a plan of more positive action. Make a list and don't hold back: The micromanaging boss fat. The fear of starting my own company fat. The "will I ever find the partner of my life?" fat. Money troubles fat. When you name it, you can tame it. By telling your True Truth, you're already removing some of your Mental Fat.

2. Create Your Power Why

What will keep you motivated when you're about to reach for that box of cookies? What's your deepest fear? Not living long enough to see your grandchildren? Being dependent on others? Being too fat to enjoy life? Whatever it is, name it. Now think about what the opposite of that fear would be for you. That's your Power Why—what you *really* want.

A Power Why always comes down to two consequences. For instance, a 45-year-old patient of mine who has high blood pressure lives for his wife and two kids and is afraid of

> "They always say time changes things, but you actually have to change them yourself."
>
> —*Andy Warhol*

losing any time with them. If he keeps making poor lifestyle choices, he'll lose his family through premature heart disease. If he chooses right, he'll keep his family by staying healthy. So his is Lose 'Em or Keep 'Em. What's your Power Why?

3. Discover What Takes You to the Dark Place and Make Different Plans

Are you a perfectionist? A ruminator? Anxious? Disappointed? Afraid of change? Once you see your vulnerabilities, you create the freedom to change them. Get a notebook and keep track of every time you go to the Dark Place and Bottom Feed. Then write down the circumstance under which each event took place. Pretty soon, you'll notice a pattern: Bottom Feeding happens when I'm dealing with my spouse or the misbehaving child; when I have a fight with my best friend; facing a messy, cluttered house; when money issues come up.

Now that you're aware, you can choose to operate at a higher level of functioning. That's where your Life Stress Scenarios come in.

4. Create a Life Stress Scenario List to Practice A²

Practice preemptive strikes. What if my father falls down the stairs and has to move in with me? What if I have a money crisis? Make a list of five potential Life Stress Scenarios in each category (Mind, Mouth, etc.) that could happen within the first 12 weeks of your Fit to Live journey. Now brainstorm one way to embrace every challenge as a golden opportunity to grow and hone your A² skills.

5. Connect to Your Spirituality

There are three words I use all the time. They come from the runner Flo-Jo: Believe. Achieve. Succeed. You have to do them in *that* order. You cannot succeed without belief. That's why it's important to find one simple way to connect to your spirituality. Make up a prayer, even if it's just a phrase, and say it once per day. Read a book of daily spiritual passages, keep a journal where you can write prayers and spiritual thoughts, go to a place of worship weekly—anything where you connect to your higher power and honor the sacred.

TO ENJOY:

If you scored a 7 to 13 on the test, just take a quick look at the "To Survive" suggestions. If you feel you have them covered, you can start here.

1. Capitalize on Your Strengths

Being Mentally Fit to Live will be easier and more enjoyable when you use your strengths. When I first met with Pat, she was a self-proclaimed perfectionist. A fourth-grade teacher, she was superb at almost everything she did—except eating right and exercising. Her chronic perfectionism fooled her into thinking she could apply the same attitude to her body as she did to her color-coded towels.

I asked her, "When a fourth-grade child is learning how to multiply, do they never once screw up a problem?"

"Oh, I get it!" she said. "I need to treat myself the way I treat my students when they're learning! I can do that!"

Stop and really look at your strengths. Are you someone who understands how to interact with people? Someone who is responsible? Goal oriented? A great dad or mom? Write five strengths. Now, like I did with Pat, ask yourself, "How can I use my strengths to make this more enjoyable?" Take your marvelous attributes and make them work for you.

2. Become a Change Agent

You're now someone who can embrace change. How about takin' it to the streets? Is there a community or civic group that could benefit from your leadership? You might be surprised what one small effort can accomplish. When I became medical director for the Race for the Cure in Washington, D.C., this amazing 5-K event had 17,000 participants. I'd just met Sharon Stone and thought, boy, if I could connect her to the event, I bet we'd get more participants, which would yield more money available for breast cancer research and education. One phone call later, she agreed; that June, we expanded to 27,000 participants. Today, our 5-K is the largest in the world, with 70,000 participants every year.

Everyone has the power to be a change agent, especially when you connect with others. People who are Mentally Fit to Live enjoy making a difference!

TO CHALLENGE:

If you scored a 14 to 20 on the test, just take a quick look at the "To Survive" and "To Enjoy" tips. If you feel you have them covered, you can start here.

1. Adopt the Rule of Seven

A friend once told me of a Native American saying: "If you haven't thought of seven ways to deal with something, your thinking is incomplete." Challenge yourself to think of seven possible healthy ways to respond to any Body Dollar binge. For instance, you reach for the cookie jar when you feel insecure. Here are seven other possible ways to respond:

1. Call a friend who will say, "You can do it!"
2. Write down all your positive attributes.
3. Remind yourself of the times you handled something well.
4. Imagine the wisest person you know telling you what to do. What does she say?
5. Feel the feeling and take positive action anyway.
6. Have a good cry and then take a walk.
7. Tell yourself it's okay to be insecure, and then use your Power Why to stay focused.

2. Become a Fearless Warrior

Write down your greatest fears: public speaking, heights, financial ruin, getting dumped by your partner, never seeing the wonders of the world, failing at your professional work. Now prioritize the items on your list, starting with the ones that would have the greatest impact on your life right now. (Scaling tall mountain peaks is not an immediate issue. However, financial ruin is.) Choose one of the top three. Let's say you choose money. Now prepare to make some changes. Assemble the people who can help you develop and execute a plan. Take small steps, because you know this issue is anxiety provoking. Acknowledge your accomplishments along the way. See that the greatest achievement is not monetary but your ability to become fearless.

3. Retreat to Grow

I conduct Peeke Week Retreats throughout the year, taking men and women into national park forests, mountains, and even the Grand Canyon, to hone their Fit to Live skills. By retreating from the constraints of everyday life, people can regroup and gain a deeper appreciation of their lives. Retreats, especially those in nature, are humbling, glorious experiences where we can expand our A^2 skills. I wish I could see every reader of this book at one of my Peeke Week Retreats! Find a retreat you might like—yoga, religious, outdoor adventure, gender specific, family oriented. Show yourself you're Fit to Live to challenge.

CHAPTER 3

Practice Safe Stress

"Let your soul stand cool and composed before a million universes."
—*WALT WHITMAN*

Raise your hand if you think that stress is at the core of your problems. Now raise your hand if you think your goal is to lead a stress-free life.

Yep, that's what I thought. If you raised your hand to either or both of those questions, you're wrong. Stress is an integral piece of life. Without stress, we would never refine our A^2 skills to survive, enjoy, and challenge ourselves.

Stress is not the problem. *Distress* is. Distress happens when we aren't managing stress well, when we associate stress with feelings of helplessness, hopelessness, and defeat. When we choose to respond to stress by becoming distressed, we go to the Dark Place. Distress is Toxic Stress, and it costs huge amounts of Body Dollars.

And Toxic Stress makes you fat. As I revealed in my books *Fight Fat After Forty* and *Body-for-LIFE for Women*, Toxic Stress leads to overeating, which leads to that Toxic Belly Fat. Stress-eating affects both genders, but women are hardest hit. Men tend to hit the

> *"If you are distressed by anything external, the pain is not due to the thing itself, but to your estimate of it; and this you have the power to revoke at any moment."*
>
> —*Marcus Aurelius Antoninus*

beer and wine under stress, while women are tearing through boxes of Girl Scout cookies and other fatty sweet treats.

Toxic Stress makes you sick and can even shorten your life. Harboring chronic Toxic Stress can lead to heart disease, poor immune function, hair loss, poor memory, diabetes, and, for women, vaginal infections and female infertility. Toxic Stress makes you grow older faster. It literally take years off your life by shortening the little caps called telemeres at the end of your chromosomes. When telemeres are shortened, cells die. The result is a rapidly advanced aging process. Groundbreaking research has discovered that women with the highest levels of perceived stress—Toxic Stress—from caring for children with chronic illness have shorter telemeres compared with low-stress women. The end result? The aging process is accelerated by a factor of *10 years*.

Centenarians—folks who live to 100 or beyond—demonstrate amazing ability to A² whatever life throws at them: death of loved ones, illness, poverty, even imprisonment in concentration camps. The reason this is so crucial can be found in our body's physiology.

⇒Our Toxic Lifestyle⇐
Welcome to the Overwhelming, Overbusy Lifestyle

"Every problem has a gift for you in its hands."
—RICHARD BACH

The stress response is hardwired. It's the same one our human ancestors had, as well as other primates. The part of our brain that's involved in the stress response, known as the limbic system, works just like that of other mammals. Neurologist Paul MacLean, MD, named this our emotional brain, concerned with feelings, instincts, eating, fighting, and sexual behavior. It's constantly scanning for "pleasant" or "painful" and "safe" or "dangerous."

When you perceive any stress at all, good or bad—a dozen roses show up mysteriously at the front door or an IRS agent comes knocking—it triggers a rush of master hormones that pour out of the brain in nanoseconds and zip over to the adrenal glands, which sit on top of each kidney. Once these glands are stimulated, two best friends—the stress hormone cortisol and the neurotransmitter norepinephrine (adrenalin)—are secreted. Together, they prepare your mind and body to do your best fight and flight response, including flooding your bloodstream with glucose, fatty acids, and triglycerides to fight, freeze like a rabbit trying not to be noticed, or run like hell.

This worked well for primal humans. Their stresses were all about life and death survival in the moment—run from big things that want to eat you, and run after the things you want to eat. The vast majority of time, it was life or death in a few moments. If a tarantula fell on your back, you ran. Thing is, that tarantula didn't cling to your back for 3 years straight. And your short, shrugging, screaming sprint burned off the glucose, fatty acids, and triglycerides that had flooded your bloodstream to begin with.

As we moved from hunters and gatherers to farmers and then industrialized workers, we worked our bodies intensely. The chemical reactions created by the stresses we encountered were burned off before they had a chance to do lasting damage. Plus, life went at a slower pace, with much less to pay attention to. There was time to "do nothing," which allowed our bodies and minds to recover.

In the past few decades, we've evolved into human "doings" that are on 24/7. The quality and quantity of the stresses in our lives have changed dramatically, but our bodies' response has remained the same for a million years. And that, dear friends, is a big part of why we're presently in so much trouble.

Fascinating FAToid

"I Can Handle This"

A typical reaction to stress is a panicked response psychologists call catastrophizing: "This is awful, and it's only going to get worse." When we forget a name and panic, for instance, we poison our brains with stress hormones and make it less possible to remember. New research shows that when people learn techniques to stop catastrophizing, their brains show greater information processing and problem-solving intelligence, even 3 years later. **Bottom line:** Practicing Safe Stress is good for body and mind.

Fascinating FAToid

What's That You Just Said?

One kind of stress scientists have identified is "concept shifting"—the stress of changing our focus from one thing to another. The average North American worker shifts concepts 10 to 20 times every hour, up to 200 times a day. **Bottom line:** A^2 it throughout the day so that you don't end up going for the ice cream "cure" at 4 p.m.

We are now constantly dealing with endless interruptions and flooded with so much information that we're paying "continuous partial attention" to everything. My friend, former Microsoft executive Linda Stone, coined this term to describe how we are all constantly scanning the environment rather than focusing on any one thing. This, say scientists, negatively affects our brain's capacity to learn and recall information later.

Americans are also working more than medieval peasants did and more than the citizens of any other industrial country—almost 9 weeks longer per year than folks in Western Europe. Work hours are up to 1,978 hours per year on average, an increase of 1 week more than in 1990, with managers and professionals increasing the most. (This is only *office* hours, so it doesn't include time worked on weekends, at home, in cars, in airplanes, or on laptops, cell phones, and e-mail.)

Many of us get no paid vacation, and more than one-third of us don't take our allotted vacation time because of "too much work." A recent study concluded that "Americans are the most vacation-starved people in the industrialized world." US workers average a little over 2 weeks of vacation per year, while Europeans average 5 to 6.

Some economists say we're working too much because as knowledge workers, what we produce is not tangible—and therefore can't be easily measured except in hours worked. So we overwork to prove our worth. That's why taking no time for yourself has become a badge of honor. Who will be at work first? Who will be out of there last?

I had a patient who looked at me the other day and told me, "Well, I took my first vacation in 5 years. And it took so long to catch up when I came back, I shouldn't have gone in the first place!" Do you play that dangerous game?

In Japan, working yourself to death is called *karoshi,* and in China, it's known as *guolaosi.* We don't have a term in English, but we probably will soon. All this work and no time off has consequences. Overwork (defined, by the way, as more than 45 hours every week—how much more are YOU doing?) is associated with an increased risk of high blood pressure, heart disease, fatigue, depression, musculoskeletal disorders, chronic infections, diabetes, and other general health complaints.

> "Expect trouble as an inevitable part of life, and when it comes, hold your head high, look it squarely in the eye, and say, 'I will be bigger than you. You cannot defeat me.'"
> —Ann Landers

Chronic stress is connected to Toxic Belly Fat Syndrome, that dangerous cluster of conditions you learned about in Chapter 1. Working long hours increases women's (but not men's) consumption of high-fat and high-sugar snacks, caffeine, and cigarettes, and decreases their exercise time. It's not more work but the stress from work that's causing these negative effects on women. Experiencing just one stressful event, like a blown deadline or important meeting, was linked for women to greater snacking on unhealthy food and fewer portions of healthy foods like fruits and vegetables.

Why do women go for the candy calm? Women produce less of the feel-good hormone serotonin than men do, and high-fat, high-sugar foods actually drive the stress hormones down. As women wean themselves off the daily hits of comfort food, there's a transition period of crabbiness followed by increased energy and calm. One of the most important things to keep in mind when it comes to stress is that the mind and body are *exquisitely* interconnected. When you get stressed out, the hormones affect *everything*. These present-day stresses collide with our primal brain physiology, and for many of us, the fight or flight mechanism, which was supposed to be for short-term life-or-death emergencies, is turned

Fascinating FAToid

Information Overload, Anyone?

The amount of information the world produces doubled between 2000 and 2003 to 5 exabytes of information yearly. Five exabytes is equivalent to 37,000 new libraries the size of the Library of Congress. **Bottom line:** We're under siege by mostly unimportant data. Prioritize so you don't get overwhelmed and pack on the pounds in response.

Fascinating FAToid
Stressed about Stress

- 62 percent of people say work has a significant impact on stress levels.
- 73 percent name money as their number one stress.
- 54 percent are concerned about the level of stress in their everyday lives.

Bottom line: Practice your A^2 every day to keep this stress from becoming distress and to prevent damage to your body.

on most of the time. The brain is specifically vulnerable. If you sectioned the areas of the brain after you had chronic elevations of cortisol day after day, week after week, what you will notice is cellular death. Meaning, we're killing our brain cells from Toxic Stress, which affects everything from our moods to our ability to feel and sense.

Chronic elevations of cortisol are toxic to every single tissue in the human body. Here are a few of the other dangerous effects:

- Higher "bad" cholesterol and lower "good" cholesterol
- Fatigue
- Ulcers
- Irritable bowel syndrome
- Depression
- Low sex drive
- Memory impairment
- Inability to concentrate or think creatively
- Hardening of the arteries
- Lack of quality and quantity of sleep
- Osteoporosis
- Inflammatory arthritis
- Alzheimer's (by impairing the brain's ability to block harmful molecules)

In my book *Fight Fat After Forty,* I describe cortisol's role in refueling appetite, thereby causing stress-eating and Toxic Belly Fat, especially in women. In response to the hunger cortisol creates, women make it a mission to go out and eat large quantities of whatever they can find. Men, on the other hand, tend to go toward alcohol under stress, which causes physical, emotional, and social problems of its own.

However stress shows up for you, it's never one episode that triggers these terribly negative effects. It's the piling up of one on top of another and lasting over time. That's why it's so hard to say, "This one thing caused this."

SOME IMPORTANT WORDS ABOUT SLEEP

Need more evidence that we need to practice Safe Stress? We can't sleep because of all the stress hormones chugging through our veins. Folks over 40 have the poorest sleep habits of any generation in history. Seventy-million of us have some kind of chronic sleep problem. The use of sleep medications has quadrupled in the past 10 years. Fifty-five percent of us now have trouble sleeping, causing problems in our relationships, driving abilities, and work performance. Women are not only more likely than men to report insomnia, but also more likely to have daytime sleepiness. They begin to have sleepless nights during menstruation, pregnancy, or menopause, then find it difficult to break poor sleep habits.

When you've got too much on your plate, you know what happens. You slice and dice those sleep hours until you're running on 4 hours of sleep. Why is this bad? Not enough sleep is associated with high blood pressure, cancer, heart attacks, irritability, and impaired thinking and judgment. Not good.

It will also put the Toxic Fat on your belly. If you sleep less than 4 hours every night,

---

THE MOOD–BELLY FAT CONNECTION

The use of antidepressants by adults nearly tripled between 1988 to 1994 and 1999 to 2000—and a majority of the users are overweight or obese. Drugs such as Effexor often cause dramatic weight gain of 30 pounds or more. Folks who are obese have a higher prevalence of all mood and anxiety disorders over their lifetimes. Which comes first—obesity or mood disorders—is not clear. But scientists estimate that one-quarter of the cases of obesity are attributable to mood disorders. If you are overweight or obese, you must honor how you're hardwired psychologically. Don't just plunge into the technical aspects of eating and exercise; you've got to improve your A^2 skills so that life stresses don't continue to derail your goal to become Fit to Live.

"Over the years, your
bodies become walking
autobiographies,
telling friends and
strangers alike of
the minor and major
stresses of your lives."
—*Marilyn Ferguson*

you're 73 percent more likely to be obese than someone who sleeps 7 to 9. Sleep deprivation actually *doubles* the risk of obesity for adults and children and is showing up in children as young as 5. Women who sleep 5 hours a night or less gain 30 percent more than those who slept 7, a greater influence than exercise or diet.

The reason is that sleeping less affects your resting metabolic rate (number of calories burned while sleeping). Plus the less you sleep, the less of the hormone leptin your body produces. Leptin helps you feel full and gets you into motion. So a lack of leptin may be causing you to eat more and move less.

Another hormone that makes you feel hungry—ghrelin—is much higher in the sleep deprived. In one study, men who got poor sleep increased their calories by 1,000 per day because they felt starved even when they weren't; they gained weight and began having the blood sugar problems found in people with pre-diabetes.

Sleep deprivation doesn't just ramp up the odds for diabetes and obesity, it can literally take your breath away. Poor sleep causes weight gain, and weight gain can cause sleep apnea, which can interrupt sleep even further. Sleep apnea is a potentially dangerous condition where you stop breathing due to the obstruction of the flow of air in your breathing passage. It's usually caused by the softening of tissue and the accumulation of fat around the tonsils acting like a lid, cutting off breathing. When you stop breathing, you wake up many times per hour without knowing it. Your body doesn't get REM (rapid eye movement) sleep, which occurs only after 90 minutes of sleep onset, so you wake up tired. Left untreated, sleep apnea can cause morning headaches, high blood pressure, memory loss, stroke, and, by triggering abnormal heartbeats and other cardiovascular difficulties, death.

Fascinating FAToid

Sugar Sweet Sleep

In research sponsored by the National Institutes of Health, men and women with type 2 diabetes had better control of their blood sugar when the duration and quality of their sleep was optimal. **Bottom line:** Sleep is rejuvenating, relaxing, and healing—a real package deal.

The treatment for sleep apnea is either surgery—only 50 percent successful—or wearing a CPAP mask while sleeping to keep your oxygen level up. My patients who are married to someone with sleep apnea usually sleep in another bedroom because the hissing of oxygen into the mask all night gives *them* sleep deprivation.

Guess what? Cut the Belly Fat, and the sleep apnea problem tends to clear up. You don't have to cut much—remove only 10 pounds, and the sleep apnea episodes reduce by 30 percent.

Getting the picture? Aren't you fed up with being fat, distressed, perpetually exhausted, and sleep deprived? Don't your funky responses to all of this Toxic Stress—overeating, drinking, smoking, drugs, social withdrawal, anger—get old? To save your life, to trim your waist, you've got to practice Safe Stress.

⇨ Fit to Live ⇦
Permission to Chill, Sir!

"For fast-acting relief, try slowing down."
—LILY TOMLIN

In many respects, life provides each and every one of us with an endless number of opportunities to practice Safe Stress. No one can do this perfectly. But you can get better and better at it. You may have crappy days—days when you scarf down three Ho-Hos because you're stressed out over a deadline at work. But you'll have more days when you A² well and instead breathe deeply or exercise through the stress instead. Ahh, now you're not only conserving Body Dollars, you're investing more into your Body Dollar bank. It's all about embracing five basic ways of thinking so you have more good days than bad.

THE FIVE FIT TO LIVE SAFE STRESS PRINCIPLES

1. Life Will Throw You Curves; Just Don't Let Them Throw You

Nothing much is a big deal. Nothing. When you remember that, you minimize health-destruction from stress. And that, as you've just learned, is a very good thing.

Fascinating FAToid

Depression-Proof Yourself

Depression is two to three times higher in people with type 2 diabetes than in the general population. The use of antidepressants by a pre-diabetic person increases their risk of developing diabetes. **Bottom line:** Start today to live the healthy Fit to Live lifestyle, and you get the big win/win—preventing or reversing type 2 diabetes, while controlling depression.

Consider this tale of distress. When I was on tour for *Body-for-LIFE for Women,* I was flying from New York to Billings, Montana. I ended up stranded at midnight in the Denver airport because of a freak hailstorm. When the announcement came, I was tired. I'd gotten up at 0-dark-hundred to do early-morning television. We'd already been diverted to another airport in Colorado. Customer service had just informed us that not only were no planes taking off that evening, but every single hotel in Denver was sold out.

While we were waiting in line, a woman next to me was exploding: "I *have* to get to Boston tonight!" she kept screaming. As I watched, she folded down to her knees and broke into hysterics, at which point, somebody behind her said, "Lady, get over it! None of us are going anywhere!" I felt so sad for her as she went from stress to distress and spent a 401k's worth of Body Dollars.

Now consider another story: A lovely 49-year-old woman had come to me to learn to manage her menopausal body transition. I was blown away as she calmly shared her life story—the discovery of kidney disease during her one and only pregnancy, the death by drowning of her only child, the extreme stress of which resulted in her going into premature menopause at 45, the car crash that threw her kidney disease into a life-threatening crisis, and her successful—thank you, God—kidney transplant. I asked her how she managed to endure. She smiled and said, "Somewhere along the line, I just accepted the ebb and flow of life. It's just not worth it to complain and fight these events. I just pick up with the help of my loved ones and keep on truckin'." Amen, and so can you.

2. Watch Out for Stress-Free Expectations

When people come to me, countless thousands over the years, and say, "Dr. Peeke, I'm just absolutely going to make it work this time, because this is a time of low stress in my life, and I don't expect any major stresses," I'm scared. Because that's not possible.

So many people get stressed because they expect things to be stress free. Then they are shocked when things are hard and proceed to self-destruct. The deal that didn't come through, the project that has deadline pressure, the traffic on the 405, the husband who becomes depressed. Each bump of life is absolutely shocking. If this is true for you,

> "Small minds are much distressed by little things. Great minds see them all but are not upset by them."
>
> —*François de La Rochefoucauld*

ask yourself if the event was truly unexpected: You married a guy with depression in his family, and he was already hospitalized twice for it. When it happens again, why the surprise?

The phone is going to ring. Did you win the lottery? Or are you going to find out that your son fell down and broke an elbow? No matter what happens, can you make it work?

One thing that helps is to add a dash of wit and humor. Can you say to yourself, "This is going to make one *hell* of a story!"? Then take a deep cleansing breath and live through the problem as best as possible.

3. Pound Out Perfection, Bring On Progress

Expecting yourself to be perfect costs tremendous amounts of Body Dollars. Perfectionism equals paralysis. Perfectionists never get anywhere, because the minute they feel they have not been "perfect," they stop dead in their tracks and go back to Bottom Feeding. Or they never begin because they are too afraid of not doing it "perfectly."

Perfectionism assumes that you can control everything. I don't want to break anyone's heart, but you can't control anything but your own response to life's challenges. There you

Fascinating FAToid

Walk Your Brain

So many of what we thought were the symptoms of aging are actually the symptoms of disuse. This is especially true for the brain. Stress management, along with memory exercises, coupled with a healthy lifestyle of good nutrition and exercise, optimizes memory and brain function. **Bottom line:** Feed your brain with nutritious foods, nurture it by practicing Safe Stress, and take it for a walk today.

Fascinating FAToid
The Weight of Stress

Men stress out about weight and get assertive about shedding pounds when they are told they have to take pills, especially those that interfere with sexual functioning. Women seek weight reduction when they become stressed enough about appearance, energy level, and poor self-esteem. **Bottom line:** Although Mars and Venus are motivated differently, the solution is still to target that Toxic Belly Fat to get Fit to Live.

are, perfectly dressed in a beautiful suit, then someone trips and dumps coffee on you. Bam—you're not perfect anymore.

Perfectionists think, "I will eat perfectly." There's no such thing. Those who are Fit to Live eat as appropriately as possible under the circumstances of a constantly changing environment. You're at the airport. What do you think they have there, Golden Door spa food? Do the best you can.

4. Heads Down for a Mini-Chill

From the moment we wake up, it's heads up for everything. We push, prod, and beat those brain cells into submission, squeezing the living daylights out of them to remember phone

Voice of Success: "Every Day, I Wake Up and Redefine Normal."

Augie Nieto, founder of Life Fitness Corp., has Lou Gehrig's disease (ALS) and a prognosis 2 to 5 years. His disease is progressing much slower because he has the Body Dollar reserve from years of Mind and Muscle Fitness.

"Ever see an EKG? It's got peaks and valleys. If it's a flat line, you're dead. Living is all about peaks and valleys. Every day, I wake up and redefine normal. I don't mourn what I can't do. I celebrate what I can. I wake up enthusiastic about all that is still out there, like having this conversation. My zest and love of life is about feeling in control. When you feel in control, you are in control of your destiny."

Voice of Success:
Recognizing Old Stress Responses

Cindy MacRae cut 42 pounds of body fat and 6 inches around her waist

"When I journaled, I realized I ate when I was overwhelmed, angry, sad, or bored. Often, I ate something and then realized I really didn't want it. Dr. Peeke calls this mindless eating. Once I became conscious of my habits, I could change my responses. When I found myself heading toward the kitchen, I'd ask, 'Are you really hungry?' I learned how to take a breath and A^2 it through the day, and literally felt the Mental Fat lightening. With my Power Why in place—being there for my wonderful family—I stopped stress-eating, built strong muscles, and recently celebrated by running the New York City marathon. My mantra now is, 'Put forth the effort, and the results will come.'"

numbers and names, crank out work documents, ruminate about the past, worry about the future, ink endless to-do lists. Ka-ching! You spend Body Dollars without replenishing your body bank account. Did it ever occur to you that your head needed rest too? As the Dalai Lama said when I heard him speak recently, "You have to disconnect to connect." You must take time to put your head down—on a pillow to nap or comfy headrest for a brief chillin'. A mini-chill.

A mini-chill is a moment woven into the fabric of your day, time to turn your stress response down. This is *so* important. People kill themselves, spend, spend, spend, spend Body Dollars 5 days a week, thinking, "Oh, I'll make it up on the weekend." Wrong. You need a slow release of mini-chills sprinkled throughout your days to be Fit to Live. I don't care if it's listening to some music, looking at a tree, staring at your belly button. Anything you want as long it's relaxing! I recommend a mini-chill for a minute or two every hour if possible.

Sometimes, we need the permission to come from the outside. That was true for my patient Naomi. When I met her, this entrepreneur was working 100 hours per week.

As a joke one day, out of sheer frustration, I whipped out my prescription pad and wrote her name on it, put the date on it, and wrote the following: "Take 6 weeks total vacation per year and time to chill daily." Then I signed it, and in the space for "refills," I put the word "eternity." Do you know that she took that home, and to this day, 12 years later, she still has it up on her bulletin board? And she's followed it too. Down four dress sizes after

Fascinating FAToid

Time Off Can Save Your Life—Literally

Men who took the most vacations were 29 percent less likely to be diagnosed with heart disease and 17 percent less likely to die over a 9-year study period than those who did not take regular vacations. **Bottom line:** Enjoy a big return and invest those vacation Body Dollars.

cutting 40 pounds and 6 inches of Toxic Belly Fat, Naomi has sustained her success because, after all, she's following doctor's orders! (And I'd like you to consider this book your very own prescription!)

5. If Not Now, *When*?

This is a special principle for all those caregivers out there who keep putting themselves at the bottom of their to-do list. Stop deferring self-care! We now know that the best caregiver, male or female, is the healthiest one. Researchers took two groups of caregivers who were taking care of chronically ill people. One group basically said, "I'm stopping everything in my life because I'm caring for this person. I'm not going to take a walk; I'm not going to eat well; I'm not going to take a break." The other, more-balanced group said, "You know something? I *have* to take care of myself if I'm going to take really good care of this person." They drew blood from both groups and challenged it with viruses and cancer cells. Guess what? The white cells in the unbalanced group were unable to fight off disease, while those in the balanced group could. When they actually followed the unbalanced caregivers over time, many ended up dying before the people that they were supposed to be taking care of! You have to include yourself in your own caring. Make your new self-care motto "If not now, *when*?" It could very well save your life.

⇨Fit to Live Essentials⇦

Using your score from the "Are You Mentally Fit to Live?" test, you'll continue to build your individual program with the tips below. As in Chapter 2, you'll begin according to your current level, master those skills, and then move on. Don't forget about the template in Appendix 2 that will help you organize your individual plan.

TO SURVIVE:

If you received a score of 0 to 6 on the test, focus your energy here first. Once you've mastered these, feel free to move up to the tips in "To Enjoy."

1. Breathe Through Stress

When you see that concrete ball of stress swingin' your way, take a slow, deep breath. Just one breath. Feels pretty good, doesn't it? When you breathe that way, you actually alter the levels and ratios of brain chemicals that calm you. Inhale for a count of three and exhale for a count of four. Enjoy that exhalation. In with the good, out with the bad.

2. Get Straight about Stress

Let's get this straight. There are two basic kinds of stress: (1) life threatening and (2) annoying but livable. Are you someone who keeps kicking in your big-time stress response (appropriate for life-threatening stresses like medical emergencies) for what should be annoying but livable stress (someone outbid you on the house you had your heart set on)? True emergencies require a serious withdrawal from the Body Dollar bank to save your life. Annoying but livable stresses should require a much smaller withdrawal. Be careful not to bankrupt your Body Dollar bank with what should be minor expenses.

3. Convert Expectations to Hope

Go back to what you consider to be some of the roughest times in your life, and look at what the stress was. Most if not all of the time, it's attached to some expectation. He never asked you to marry him. Your kid doesn't reciprocate with the same level of love you have for him/her. You never expected to have a heart attack at the age of 45.

Clinging to expectations takes you to the "this isn't fair" place. News flash: In life, fairness is a moot point. It is what it is. Replace expectations with hope. Hope leaves open the option that anything is possible.

Try it right now. Write down the stresses in your life that you have a tendency to turn into distress, or Toxic Stress. These are the challenges that really bug you deep inside. Start with the neighbor who plowed through

> "Turn down the volume in your life and turn up the silence."
> —*Maria Shriver*

your prize bushes with his lawn mower. Instead of getting steamed, or blaming, or stewing, just say, "I hope, after his apology, he doesn't do it again." Or, instead of remaining bitter with your remote child, say, "I hope my kid appreciates all I have done one day," and move on. Start hoping rather than expecting.

4. Use It, Then Sleep on It

Never underestimate the power of sleep to trim your belly. Be sure to get enough—on average, 7 hours a night (kids and teens need more!). Naps are okay, but nighttime sleep is best. Try to go to sleep and get up at the same time. Just as your other daily routines need to be ritualized, so does rest. Stay away from caffeine past noon. Create a relaxing routine—warm bath, soft music, reading for pleasure. Keep the bedroom cool, dark, and quiet. And get off that TV, computer, and Crackberry an hour before sleep!

If you have chronic trouble sleeping, you may be taking your stresses to bed with you. That's a crowd you don't need. Rather than run for a pill, do at least 30 minutes of brisk cardio exercise earlier in the day. Listen to a meditation tape or CD. Avoid the national news before you hit the sack. Stash a notebook and paper in your nightstand, and write down your worries rather than allow them to keep you awake. All these measures can help improve the quality of your sleep.

5. Be Sure to Get Your Mini-Chills

They say that stress is a disease of time deficiency. But enjoyment of anything in life involves savoring the moment. Whether you're tasting a crème brulée or watching a flock of birds take flight, rushing through destroys the enjoyment. Every day, schedule in no less than 10 minutes to go to a quiet place—the closet or bathroom are perfectly acceptable, having used them many times myself!—and choose to either sit and close your eyes, or savor an experience—drink that cup of green tea, listen to calming music, read something that is enjoyable to you. You'll be amazed how such a small moment of bliss can neutralize so much stress.

TO ENJOY:

If you scored a 7 to 13 on the test, just take a quick look at the "To Survive" suggestions. If you feel you have them covered, you can start here.

1. Burn It Off

How about a win/win/win? Get up and dance. Crank up the CD player, radio, or MP3 player and let it rip. Whether it's 50 Cent or Tony Bennett, you'll burn off Toxic Belly Fat and distress and have fun. Walk it off, run it off, swim it off. Exercise releases pent-up energy and burns off the stress hormones that otherwise can lead to weight gain, sleep troubles, and/or fights with loved ones. Did you know that overweight, postmenopausal women who exercise in the morning experience less difficulty falling asleep and better-quality sleep than evening exercisers? Sign me up! Your feel-good hormones—beta endorphins and serotonin—are now officially in overdrive.

2. Lean On 'Em

To increase your enjoyment and relieve stress, how about putting in the work to cultivate better relationships? Whip out that list of friends and family members you haven't called in a while. Grab the phone, hit the e-mail, but make it happen. People who maintain at least two or three meaningful relationships (friends, family) heal twice as fast from medical conditions (heart attacks, cancer) than people who have none. Maintaining those friendships increases your odds for living long and well at least threefold.

3. Laugh a Lot

It's humanly impossible to laugh joyfully and feel Toxic Stress at the same time. Did you know that kids laugh 300 times a day and the typical adult laughs less than 10 times a day? Find sources of great humor and chuckle away. I love old clips from *Saturday Night Live*. I read Mark Twain's witty wisdom and can't get enough of Robin Williams and Lily Tomlin. Check out www.humortop.com for some great sources of humor.

TO CHALLENGE:

If you scored a 14 to 20 on the test, just take a quick look at the "To Survive" and "To Enjoy" tips. If you feel you have them covered, you can start here.

1. Best the Beast

Everyone has one or two absolutely ass-kicking stresses in their lives that constantly haunt them. Now it's time to face the challenge. When I first met my patient Johari, she was a beautiful but distressed African American woman, 42 years old and 50 pounds heavier

> "Adopting the right attitude
> can convert a negative
> stress into a positive one."
> —*Dr. Hans Selye*

than she should be. Her inability to shed pounds was mystifying to her. She loved to exercise, but she lost out to Almond Fudge every night. When I asked her about the Dark Place, she tearfully revealed that she was only a dissertation away from her PhD in economics. She'd let stresses interrupt achieving her goal. And every night, when she was tired and vulnerable, the PhD beast showed up, stirring up her stress hormones and driving her to the ice cream solution. I told her to face off with the beast. She finally did, and after 2 years, I can now refer to her as Dr. Rashad. By Cutting her Mental Fat, she also cut the 50 pounds of Toxic Belly Fat. Identify your own beasts and cut your own fat!

2. Be a Guiding Light

How could you be a guiding light for people who are overwhelmed with Toxic Stress? One of my patients helped calm a woman who was terrified of flying. Smiling and laughing, she got the woman's mind off the turbulence. Ask yourself right now, who could I help, and how might I start? Think of the nurses and psychologists who travel to communities around the world to offer their services when natural disasters occur. Perhaps in your own neighborhood, there's an elderly or disabled person who could really use your friendship and skills. This challenge is a special one. It's part of the web of life. You give and you get.

PART 2

Mouth: Are You Nutritionally Fit to Live?

"If it comes through a car window,
it's not food."
—FORMER ARKANSAS GOVERNOR MIKE HUCKABEE

This section addresses the question, Am I Nutritionally Fit to Live? To Survive, to Enjoy, to Challenge—and to save my life? By the time you're done with this section, you'll understand the bottom-line basics to build and nourish the muscles that will increase Body Dollar reserves. Being Nutritionally Fit will also help save your life by trimming that Toxic Belly Fat and reducing your risk for heart disease, diabetes, and cancer.

Being Nutritionally Fit to Live is all about maximizing the quality, quantity, and frequency of your eating. That's why I've devoted a chapter to each. After we've covered those fundamentals, you'll learn the secrets for achieving and maintaining weight reduction. I'll give you a hint—all healthy diets work. What we do is add the Fit to Live principles to make them stick for life.

As you read through, you'll see that the Mental Fat you've cut in the previous section reveals a powerful voice in your head to overcome the TV chip commercials and malls reeking of Cinnabon fumes.

To begin, find out your current Nutritionally Fit to Live level:

1. Describe your normal eating pattern:
   a. No time for meals: You tend to graze whenever and wherever you can. Fast-food restaurant workers know you by name.
   b. Hitting it mostly right: Usually you eat three healthy meals a day.
   c. Eating the right amount of the right things: You eat three modest healthy meals and two or three appropriate-size healthy snacks.

2. You've just had a day from hell. The boss hated your report, you just found out that your checking account is overdrawn, and your kid is flunking Spanish. So you:
   a. Stuff your face with as many Doritos as you can.
   b. Allow yourself a modest indulgence like a small piece of dark chocolate.
   c. Comfort yourself with a good book, a soak in the tub, or a run.

3. Do you eat breakfast every day?
   a. Absolutely.
   b. Most days you'll grab a bran muffin or have a bowl of cereal.
   c. Yeah, right. You're too busy racing out the door to work to be bothered. Besides, it's a great way to take or keep weight off.

4. How many alcoholic drinks do you have each week?
   a. 0 or 1.
   b. 2 to 6.
   c. Who's counting? But if you had to, it's 7 or more.

5. If you live with other people, how often do you sit down and eat as a family?
   a. You're off in all directions, so almost never unless you're going through the drive-through together.
   b. At least one meal a day, usually breakfast or dinner.
   c. Sporadically; more likely to happen on weekends.

6. When it comes to food labels you:
   a. Glance at the front of the package. Who can understand those darn things on the back anyway? Besides, you love the taste. That's why you're buying it.

    b. Scan the Nutrition Facts for fat or sodium levels.

    c. Make purchases based on both Nutrition Facts and ingredients.

7. Your work is full of food challenges—bowls of candy, the vending machine, pizza and fried food in the cafeteria—or you are a Road Warrior and often find yourself at the airport or minibar with similar choices. You:

    a. Look for the least bad thing—like salad or nuts.

    b. Eat whatever is there and hate yourself later.

    c. Keep healthy snacks and emergency food like power bars in your briefcase so you can have healthy alternatives.

8. How many servings of fruits and vegetables do you eat each day?

    a. Do french fries count? If not, you'd guess 0 to 2, but you're not quite sure what a serving size is anyway.

    b. 3 to 6.

    c. You can't get enough—7 to 10.

9. What's the most common beverage in your day?

    a. A good balance of water, lots of herbal tea, and up to 3 cups of caffeinated coffee or tea.

    b. Mostly caffeinated sodas and coffee. You singlehandedly keep Starbuck's and Coca-Cola in business.

    c. A lot of water, but also some carbonated and caffeinated drinks.

10. It's Thanksgiving and you're at your mother-in-law's house. You:

    a. Stuff yourself with whatever there is. After all, it's a special occasion. Plus you don't want to make waves.

    b. Take small servings of the fatty meats, larger servings of whatever vegetables are offered, and exclaim you are "too full from all that wonderful food" to indulge in dessert.

    c. Arrive bearing gifts! Bring a vegetable tray with low-fat dip, salad, or a colorful fruit platter or other healthy food. Even if *they* won't touch the stuff, you'll be covered!

Scoring:

For each Mouth question, match your answer to the proper score.

1. a, 0; b, 1; c, 2   6. a, 0; b, 1; c, 2
2. a, 0; b, 1; c, 2   7. a, 1; b, 0; c, 2
3. a, 2; b, 1; c, 0   8. a, 0; b, 1; c, 2
4. a, 2; b, 1; c, 0   9. a, 2; b, 0; c, 1
5. a, 0; b, 2; c, 1   10. a, 0; b, 1; c, 2

Add up your score for the 10 questions and check the key below.

0 to 6: Fit to Survive. Although you're trying, you're still asleep at the meal. You need to pay more attention to simple basics here. Let food be your medicine cabinet of natural disease fighters. These are the Body Dollar reserves of nutrients you need to prevent as well as treat both physical and mental conditions. If you've gained more than 15 pounds as you move through middle age, your risk of diabetes has doubled or tripled. This is especially true if the fat you've gained is Toxic Belly Fat. However, if you lose more than 10

Bottom-Line Results from Becoming Nutritionally Fit to Live to Enjoy

■ You'll be nutritionally fueled for optimal mental and physical performance—to survive, enjoy, or to meet life's challenges.

■ You'll stop spending precious Body Dollars feeling hopeless and being hard on yourself, and instead feel empowered and in control of your healthy eating habits.

■ In combination with exercise, you'll shed your Toxic Belly Fat and reduce your waist size to the normal range (women, less than 35 inches; men, less than 40 inches).

■ You'll be able to maintain a healthy body composition (bone, fat, muscle) for life.

■ You'll reduce blood sugar and cholesterol levels.

■ You'll reduce the risk of many cancers (breast, colon) as well as dementia.

■ You'll slow the aging process, maintaining healthier skin, shinier hair, and stronger bones.

■ You'll feel fearless and able to A^2 it through any nutritional challenge.

pounds, you will cut your risk of diabetes by half. You need to increase the quality and frequency of your eating, while decreasing the total quantities. This is to eliminate that life-threatening Toxic Belly Fat and to become Nutritionally Fit to Live. Your chances of living long and well could be significantly improved.

7 to 13: Fit to Enjoy. You're banking good Body Dollar reserves listening and heeding the advice of trusted sources of healthy lifestyle information in your life. By achieving your objectives at least 80 percent of the time, you're feeling energized, and your body composition shows it. You're also building a strong biological base for prevention of the most common causes of death and disability. Even if you experience one of these conditions, you'll be able to adapt and adjust more expeditiously because you have those precious Body Dollar reserves saved up and ready for withdrawal. You have half the chance of getting heart disease or diabetes that a woman with a waist circumference of over 35 inches or a man with a waist circumference of over 40 inches has. Your chances of living long and well are excellent. You're living the Fit to Live life.

14 to 20: Fit to Challenge. You're staying on top of the ever-changing landscape of nutrition science and healthy living. If you get the alert to make change, you scope it out, make sure your trusted resources agree, and then, without any loss of time, you take action. Your Body Dollar reserves are overflowing with antioxidants, minerals, and vitamins. People like you, who eat five or more servings of fruit and vegetables a day, have been found to have about a 25 percent lower risk of cardiovascular disease and all-cause mortality in a given time period compared with people who eat fewer than five servings a day. Those who eat more than five servings a day have been found to have an even lower risk.

Your daily goal is met more than 90 percent of the time. You are a master at adapting and adjusting to dietary challenges in your daily life. Your chances of living long and well are optimal.

CHAPTER 4

Quality: What Are You Supposed to Eat?

"Tell me what you eat, and I will tell you what you are."
—ANTHELME BRILLAT-SAVARIN

D o you spend your days walking around in a food trance, mindlessly eating and drinking whatever you can lay your hands on? Every now and then, you snap out of your coma and go on a wellness binge and "do better" until a life stress hits and then, boom, you're back into your trance. It's time to stop zoning out on what you're eating and learn the simple ways you can ramp up the quality of what you're eating. In this chapter, you'll learn about what kinds of food will keep you fueled for optimal mental and physical performance, the keys to the Fit to Live lifestyle.

⇒Our Toxic Lifestyle⇐
Too Much of a Good Thing

"It's amazing how pervasive food is. Every second commercial is for food. There are 20-foot-high hamburgers up on billboards."
—ADAM SCOTT

We love sugar. Scientists speculate that we developed a love for sweetness because most of the sweet foods (berries) we ate early on were safe foods that nourished and didn't kill us. Others say our sweet tooth is naturally inborn and that we will suckle because breast milk contains lactose, a form of sugar. Either way, we're born with a love for sugar.

We also love fat. Fat had to be tasty because we needed it for survival. More often than not, there were long periods of time between antelopes. And because fat tasted so good, we ate lots of it. We stored it on our bodies and used it as fuel to keep us alive until the next big meal. We're hardwired to do this. Without that hardwiring, we'd be dead.

Since primitive times, nothing about this scenario has changed. Over time, we began growing food and keeping animals, which gave us much more food security. For the first time, humans began to eat much more highly caloric food—cream and bread, which are more calorically dense than berries. But we still had to labor physically hard to make the cream and the bread, and it still wasn't plentiful enough that we were having fourths and

Fascinating FAToid
Drowning in Sugar

Marshmallows were invented by the Egyptians and reserved for gods and royalty. Today, Americans buy 90 million pounds of marshmallows each year, about the same weight as 1,286 gray whales. How about Jell-O? Worldwide sales are 1,134,239 packages a day, or 13 boxes per second. One half-cup serving has 19 grams of sugar. **Bottom line:** If you buy mountains of refined sugar, you wear mountains of fat.

fifths. Mom might make an apple pie, with lots of sugar and fat. But it took her all day. And likely we had eight or nine siblings. We were happy to get one piece, let alone two. Food had real value. We savored that one serving. That's all we got.

Our hardwiring for sugar and fat worked for us until our environment changed. Now, we're scoring antelopes and apple pies all day long. And we're wearing them all over our body, mostly in our bellies.

The problem began in the 20th century as family farms disappeared and corporations took over the production of food on a mass scale, creating what's now known as agribusiness. With improved machinery, fertilizers, and pesticides, the result was large quantities of inexpensive food. As the capacity to grow food expanded, more and more of it became processed; today, it's a $3.3 trillion industry worldwide.

What does *processed* mean anyway? It means it's been diced, sliced, canned, packaged, and combined, with preservatives added to increase shelf life and chemicals added to improve flavor lost as it's grown in one place and then shipped across the globe. And food manufacturers aren't dumb. They understand our hardwired preference for high-sugar, high-fat foods, and they're only too happy to oblige in the products they create.

These products are not food. They are science fair projects.

When you eat a pint of ice cream, you know you're getting a boatload of sugar. But what about something as basic as crackers? In the past, crackers were made from:

o Flour
o Water
o Baking soda
o Salt

Compare that with today's Wheat Thins:

o Enriched flour
o Soybean oil
o Defatted wheat germ
o Sugar
o Corn starch
o High-fructose corn syrup

o Salt
o Corn syrup
o Monoglycerides
o Barley malt syrup
o Leavening
o Vegetable color

Notice anything? Besides the fat and chemicals, they have four kinds of sugar. Four. This is typical—the vast majority of the processed foods out there have added sugars. There's sugar in your ketchup. Sugar is even added to McDonald's french fries to give them extra crispness.

> "He who does not mind his belly will hardly mind anything else."
> —*Samuel Johnson*

Talk about the sweet life! Americans now eat 114 pounds of sugar per year. That's over ¼ pound per person per day. Sugar has gone from 11 percent of our diet in 1978 to 16 percent today, and for teens, it's as high as 20 percent. In calories, we're up to 500 calories a day in sugar, one-quarter to one-third of the total recommended calorie intake for most folks.

All this added sugar has a priming effect on our bodies: If we eat something sugary, we'll want more sugar. That's great for the food industry but disastrous for our bellies, especially for anyone who has an addiction, which is highly correlated to sugar cravings. (More on the addiction-sugar connection in the next chapter.) Besides creating Toxic Belly Fat, sugar has been linked to hyperactivity and emotional distress in teens, especially among those drinking four or more soft drinks a day.

WE'RE WEARING ALL THESE SUGARS

When I say sugar, you probably think about the white stuff made from sugar cane or beets. But there are all kinds of other sweeteners that operate the same way, turning into glucose in your bloodstream. You'll see the following words on the labels of processed foods. But it all comes down to large quantities of empty sweet calories that are expanding our waistlines.

High-fructose corn syrup

Corn syrup

Corn syrup solids

Sucrose

Dextrose

Fructose

Brown sugar

Fruit juice concentrates or any
    variation: apple juice concentrate,
    pear juice concentrate, etc.

Honey

Molasses

Maltose

Maple syrup

"When I buy cookies, I just eat four and throw the rest away. But first, I spray them with Raid so I won't dig them out of the garbage later. Be careful, though, because that Raid really doesn't taste that bad."

—*Janette Barber*

Before you go to the shame place, it's important to remember that when we scarf down all this sugar and fat in processed foods, we're just doing what we were programmed to do. One fascinating study of monkeys is the embodiment of what's happened to us. These monkeys naturally covered 10 miles a day in Africa, eating berries and leaves wherever they could. Until a resort was built nearby. Suddenly they sat all day in the trees above the garbage piles, feasting on custard and lamb bones. They weren't stupid—being primal, their number one directive was to easily access tasty food to stay alive. The result? Our primal pals developed heart disease, diabetes, and Toxic Bellies, and died prematurely.

Sound familiar? Consider the nutritional environment we've created for ourselves:

o Candy, soda, pizza, and other snacks now compete with nutritious meals in 9 out of 10 schools.

o In the '70s, we drank twice as much milk as soda. Now we drink three times more soda than milk.

o One-third of all vegetables eaten in the United States are french fries, potato chips, and iceberg lettuce. Fifty-seven percent of homemade dinners in the United States don't even include vegetables.

o In 1960, the typical American ate 4 pounds of fries and 81 pounds of fresh potatoes. In 2006, 30 pounds of fries and 49 fresh potatoes. That's four orders of fries per week!

Fascinating FAToid

Hold the Dog

Americans consume nearly 16 billion hot dogs each year—that's 70 per person. Studies have linked hot dogs to colon cancer—their preservatives contain compounds that can cause your DNA to mutate and raise your chances of getting cancer. **Bottom line:** Anyone up for roasted peanuts at the ballgame and grilled chicken at the barbecue?

- One-third of all potatoes grown now end up as fries.
- Americans ate more than 3.1 billion pounds of chocolate in 2001, almost half the world's production.
- We go through 2 billion gallons of ice cream a year—49 million scoops. The money we spend on ice cream—$20 billion—is more than the budget of NASA.

⇒Fit to Live⇐
You Have a Right to Quality Food

"You don't have to cook fancy or complicated masterpieces—just good food from fresh ingredients."
—JULIA CHILD

Your Fit to Live body needs to be nourished with high-quality foods that will help you bank Body Dollars and sustain you over the long haul. There are all kinds of simple healthy options; it's your job to A^2 it to what works best for you. Rather than give you what-to-eat whiplash—coffee, good or bad? wine, good or bad?—I'm going to lay down some bottom-line principles and the Fit to Live Essentials. (Then to make this super simple, in Appendix 2, you will find a week's worth of menus for meat eaters and vegetarians.)

THE FIVE FIT TO LIVE FOOD PRINCIPLES

1. Never Eliminate an Entire Food Group

Our bodies need healthy, whole fit macronutrients: carbohydrates, fats, and protein to sustain them over time. Period.

There are experiments that show that if you feed a warm-blooded mammal, like a rat, a normal balanced diet of rat chow with high-quality carbs, fat, and protein, and then take one of those macronutrients out—it doesn't matter which—the rat will not eat it. The rat smells a rat. How come we can't?

Our bodies need all three in the right proportions. Here's my formula:

20 to 30 Percent Fit Protein

I disagree with the current USDA recommendations of 15 percent. Assuming you have normal kidney and liver function, you need 20 to 30 percent protein to become Fit to Live. Protein is key to being lean and strong. Protein helps you feel full and fight carb cravings and enables you to build strong muscles. Fit proteins are lean meats, fish, chicken, and turkey; low- or fat-free dairy products (yogurt, cheese, milk); nuts (almonds, walnuts, cashews, reduced-fat peanut butter); and beans, such as kidney beans, chickpeas, lentils, etc. When you choose red meat, be sure it really is lean—flank steak, boneless pork loin, etc. And be sure it's not every day, because even the leanest is not as lean as the other options.

40 to 60 Percent Fit Carbs

Forget the five-servings-of-vegetables-a-day thing. Eat an unlimited amount of nonstarchy veggies, followed by four or five servings of fruit and two to four of whole grains. How come? Because these fit carbs are high in fiber, vitamins, and minerals and low in calories. Fiber has been shown to help stop the development of diabetes, high blood pressure, and heart disease and reduce your risk of obesity. Fruit and veggie intake will also improve the health of your bones, no matter what your age.

What's a starchy veggie? Beans (but not green or wax beans), peas, corn, and potatoes. Although these four vegetable categories are nutritious, they are much higher in calories. All others, munch away—and go for as many bright colors as you can. People who eat the widest variety of vegetables with the deepest colors have been shown to live longer and have the least amount of dementia and Alzheimer's, because the deeper the color, the richer and higher the level of antioxidants. Antioxidants are substances that destroy free radicals, which are oxygen molecules in the bloodstream that play a part in the development of cancer, heart disease, osteoporosis, and Alzheimer's. This is especially true for

---

NUTS ABOUT NUTS

I'm a giant nut fan. How come? They're a good source of fiber, fit fats, antioxidants, and minerals. And they may have other health benefits. Walnuts, for instance, have been shown to reduce bad cholesterol and help arteries stay healthy. Two servings of almonds a day helps women feel full and maintain a stable weight. Nuts are also easy to eat and can go anywhere, so they make the perfect snack.

Fascinating FAToid

Trans Fat Red Alert

You've probably heard that trans fats are not good for you. But guess what? They could be directly responsible for the size of your belly. It turns out that eating trans fats causes a redistribution of fat to your waist, resulting in Toxic Belly Fat. **Bottom line:** Avoid trans fats like the plague.

veggies that are deep red or orange, like tomatoes and butternut squash. They are rich in lycopene, which is very highly correlated with longevity and a decrease in dementia.

And don't forget foods rich in folate. This B vitamin is a powerhouse of protection against birth defects, heart disease, cancer, and dementia. Cooked lentils, black beans, spinach, asparagus, mustard greens, and raw broccoli are terrific sources of folate. When I think of folate, I think of the famous nun study when folate was discovered to stave off the ravages of Alzheimer's disease in the sisters. My favorite quote was that of Sister May Aloysius Wieser, who said, "Ever since the sisters heard about Dr. Snowden's folate findings, they've been making a beeline for the salad bar." Amen, sister!

When picking fruit, remember that the vitamins and fiber are great for you, but they're highly concentrated in fructose, a natural sugar. Just be careful with calorically dense fruit like berries and grapes. Make sure to stick to ½ to 1 cup at a time, no more.

20 to 30 Percent Fit Fats

Your body needs some fat. One reason is that many vitamins (A, D, E, K) and cancer-fighting compounds are fat-soluble, meaning there has to be fat in what you're eating for them to be absorbed. Adding avocado (one of the few veggies with fat) to a salad, for instance, means that you will absorb 4.4 times as much lycopene and 2.6 times as much beta-carotene as eating a salad without. If you stick to the ratios I suggest, you'll have enough fat but not too much.

Of the 20 to 30 percent, no more than 10 percent should be saturated fat and absolutely no trans fats. Trans fats are made from partially hydrogenated fats. They are as bad for your heart—and perhaps worse—than saturated fats. As of 2006, manufacturers must report on food labels when they are being used. Look for the words "partially hydrogenated" or "trans fat" and steer clear. Except for in select areas, restaurants aren't (yet) required to report and do use them a lot, especially in fried foods. If it's fried, count on trans fats unless you're told otherwise.

TIPS FOR EATING MORE WHOLE GRAINS

Eating two to four servings of whole grains a day can cut your risk of heart disease, stroke, and diabetes 20 to 36 percent. They also reduce your blood pressure and help you eat less because they're bulky. Here are some ideas for eating more of them:

✔ Substitute half the white flour with whole wheat in a recipe.

✔ Buy 100 percent whole grain bread or whole wheat pita for sandwiches and whole wheat flour tortillas instead of white.

✔ Try brown rice—there are kinds that cook in 20 minutes (such as Uncle Ben's) just like white; check the label.

✔ Cook whole wheat instant couscous—ready in 3 minutes.

✔ Have instant oatmeal instead of your regular sugary cereal.

✔ Substitute quinoa, barley, or bulgur for white rice, potatoes, or pasta.

I call the fats that are good for you fit fats. These include olive oil, canola oil, fats from nuts, omega fatty acids from fish, and coconut oil. Yes, you heard right. It turns out that coconut oil—in appropriate quantities—is actually one of the best oils you can use for heart health.

Note that I'm giving you a range in each category. What you eat in one will determine the ratio of the others so that it always adds up to 100 percent. In Chapter 5, you'll learn more specifically about quantities, and in Chapter 6, about how often you should be eating, as well as how to eat in these ratios on the go. For now, here's an easy way to envision what a Fit to Live meal looks like: Picture a large dinner plate. Now, on three-quarters of the plate, imagine a variety of raw and cooked veggies. On the remaining quarter, place a bit of lean protein and some whole grain or fruit. Keep that image in your head, and you'll automatically eat the Fit to Live way.

2. If It's White, It's Not Right

Where did all this white food come from anyway? Simple. Take perfectly healthy whole grains and strip them of their nutrients in a processing plant—voilà, light white stuff like pasta, rice, so-called "multigrain" bread. This white stuff has far less nutritive value than what these foods started as—whole grains.

As much as possible, eliminate anything made with white sugar or white starches, such as white bread and rice, processed pasta, and white potatoes. They're simply empty calories. Whole grains provide our friend fiber, as well as precious vitamins, minerals, and even some protein. Fiber helps slow the rate at which your body turns food into glucose. Food made with white flour or sugars, on the other hand, speed glucose into the bloodstream, resulting in a crash and burn as your blood sugar soars and then plummets. You end up with a ravenous appetite, eat too much, and gain Toxic Belly Fat, consequently increasing your risk of diabetes and heart disease. (There's even new evidence that people who eat white bread the most often are the most overweight.)

That being said, nobody will die if you have a doughnut every so often. Having a treat can be a healthy pleasure. Just make sure you're not eating these things every day—then it's not a treat, it's a weight-gaining staple. Instead, really savor your occasional treat and balance it with better foods and more movement throughout the rest of the day. Forty-five minutes of walking after a high-fat meal, for instance, has been shown to reverse the damage to your arteries of what you just ate.

Voice of Success: "If You Can't Do the Time, Don't Do the Crime!"

Lois and Scott Ewing, and teenage son Zack, removed 25 (Lois), 40 (Scott), and 50 (Zack) pounds

"We feel great! We totally changed our diet using Dr. Peeke's formula. What really helped was understanding that food is fuel for your metabolism, and you should eat something that not only tastes good but is good for you. In the middle of getting fit, we had to cope in a 10-week period with both Scott and Zack having surgery. What really helped us stay on track was Dr. Peeke's slogan, 'If you can't do the time, don't do the crime.' Want that cheeseburger? Go ahead and eat it as long as you eat the right way before and after and do the workouts to earn the privilege. We used that idea when we celebrated our 10th wedding anniversary. We ate what we wanted, split a dessert, and even had champagne."

3. Eat Real Food, Not Science-Fair Projects

As you've learned, there's too much sugar and, often, too much fat in most processed food. In addition, it is often stripped of micronutrients. Plus, a lot of it tastes really bizarre. Remember those flavorless fat-free snacks that were all the rage in the early '90s? Those little fudge brownie fat-free, all-sugar cookies that looked like hockey pucks? Did you ever read the side label? It looks like a biochemistry experiment. Opt for whole foods instead.

Listen to your body and demand *the real deal*. The higher the quality of your food, the higher the quality of your body. You know the saying—you are what you eat.

Go organic. It's lovely to have organic if you have the wallet that goes with it. Organic produce has higher levels of nutrients such as vitamin C and iron and less nitrates (a poison). But it's far better for your health to eat that apple than it is to avoid it because of it being nonorganic. Plus, "organic" is a slippery thing. Supposedly, it means that the food is free of most chemical pesticides and fertilizers, antibiotics, hormones, and genetic engineering. But a former chairman of the National Organics Standards board claims that there has been no enforcement of organic laws by the FDA. Also, as the market for organics grows—66 percent of the population buys "organic" at least some of the time and even Wal-Mart is getting into the market—many foods are grown in places like China and Brazil where standards are even more difficult to monitor.

Plus, as big business gets into the act, they're doing all kinds of weird things. Organic milk, for instance, is now being produced by cows that are fed organic grain in 5,000-head feedlots in the desert. That means the milk is deficient in beta-carotene and fit fats that come from cows eating grass. But it's "organic" because what the cows eat is. And note the words, "free of most chemicals." I'm sorry, but there is not an acre of arable land in the United States that hasn't been tainted with chemicals (industrial agriculture is the largest polluter). So organic is only an order of magnitude. The bottom line: If you can afford it, buy organic products. But no matter what fruits and veggies you buy, scrub 'em really well.

Fascinating FAToid

Poor Fuel Equals Poor Performance

A British study found that children who eat sugary snacks for breakfast have the reaction times of a 70-year-old when tested later. **Bottom line:** Refined sugar speeds up the aging process.

> ## BUY LOCAL
>
> Consider shopping at your local farmer's market. Because it has not traveled far distances, their produce has stronger colors and tastes and is fresher. Much is organic. To find yours, go to www.ams.usda.gov/farmersmarkets or www.localharvest.org.

Choose deep-water fish. Fish are also tricky. Fish are a magnificent source of protein as well as omega-3 fatty acids, which can cut the risk of dying from a heart attack by 36 percent. (More on that later.) However, my guess is that in only 10 to 15 years, every wild fish will be significantly tainted with mercury, PCBs, or other pollutants. Farmed fish are not the answer—they are often fed the guts of other fish, so they have an even greater concentration of toxins.

That doesn't mean you should give up fish altogether. As I write, a panel of experts has just come out with a report saying that the benefits still outweigh the risks. My recommendation is to eat wild fish two or three times a week, especially deep-ocean fish like salmon. Young children and pregnant or nursing women or those who may be pregnant should never eat shark, swordfish, or king mackerel and should choose light tuna canned in water, not albacore, but not more than once a week. Then take omega-3 supplements as suggested in the chart on pages 76 and 77, which are taken from fish but have all the chemicals filtered out.

4. Be Sensible with Supplements

The word *supplement* means just that. You should be enriching an already healthy nutritional intake. Supplements never take the place of whole foods. If you are eating in the ratios I suggest, here are my supplement recommendations. Take a good multivitamin, starting in the teenage years, to help prevent cancer, osteoporosis, and heart disease; it will help you remain Alert and Vertical. Go for a brand that has gender- and/or age-specific formulas—like Rainbow, Enzymatic Therapy, Centrum, or Nature-Made. Check to see if your selection has the amounts of the vitamins and minerals below. If not, use additional supplements to come up to the recommended amounts. Try not to overshoot my recommendations, especially with the really expensive and wild combinations of higher-dose vitamins and minerals that often come laced with a concoction of herbals.

RECOMMENDED DOSAGES OF SUPPLEMENTS

SUPPLEMENT	AMOUNT	ADDITIONAL INFORMATION
Water-Soluble Vitamins		
Thiamin	2 mg	—
Riboflavin	2 mg	—
Niacin	15 mg	A small risk exists for skeletal muscle pain and breakdown for those taking the combination of larger amounts of niacin and statin drugs. Check with your doctor.
Vitamin B_6	2 mg	—
Vitamin B_{12}	2.4 mcg*	—
Folate	800 mcg	Can also be listed as folic acid, folicin, or vitamin B_9
Biotin	30 mcg	—
Pantothenic acid	5 mg	—
Vitamin C	400 mg	Reduce this to 100 mg a day from supplements if you're taking a statin drug (for example, Zocor, Lipitor, Pravachol, or Crestor). Vitamin C at this level may act to increase the effectiveness of statins.
Fat-Soluble Vitamins		
Vitamin A	100 percent as beta-carotene and no more than 2,500 IU*	—
Vitamin D	1,000 IU if you're under 60, 1,500 IU over 60	This is above the USDA recommendation, but compelling research suggests that higher supplementation can help prevent a host of chronic diseases.
Vitamin E	50 IU of mixed tocopherols	—
Vitamin K	80 mcg	—

SUPPLEMENT	AMOUNT	ADDITIONAL INFORMATION
Minerals		
Calcium	1,000 to 1,500 mg	—
Magnesium	400 mg	—
Selenium	200 mcg	—
Zinc	15 mg	—
Iron	18 mg premenopausal women; 8 mg men and postmenopausal women	—
Iodine	150 mcg	—
Additional Supplements If You're Over 40 Years Old		
Coenzyme Q_{10}	100 to 200 mg	Has been shown to help promote heart health, and new research is being done showing that it may help prevent and treat Parkinson's and possibly dementia.
Omega-3 fatty acids	1,000 mg in the morning	If you've got a family history of heart disease or already developed high blood pressure or high cholesterol, I recommend 2,000 mg.

* Mcg: micrograms; IU: international units

I discourage taking too many supplements because we don't know the effects of the combination of these substances. We also don't know the effects of taking one substance in food in isolation from others. For example, folks used to say to take boatloads of beta-carotene. But then scientists discovered that it actually increased the incidence of lung cancer in smokers. There are a lot of different carotenoids—like 30 to 50—in vegetables such as carrots, and beta-carotene is just one of them. They're meant to be together.

5. What You Drink Matters Too

Women should be having three quarts of fluids a day, men four, and both even more in hot weather when you're active. In the purest of worlds, the fluid you should be drinking is water or herbal tea.

> ## WANT TO KNOW WHAT YOU'RE EATING?
>
> Go to www.nutritiondata.com to find a food composition analysis for thousands of foodstuffs, both fresh and processed, including many fast-food items. You can find ingredients, calories, percentages of fats and proteins, and more.

Beware the soda can. Whatever you do, limit your intake of sugar sodas. One can a day may work out to an extra 15 pounds around your belly at the end of a year. The average American now drinks 54 gallons of soda a year—that works out to 575 of the 12-ounce cans. And guess how much sugar is in each can? Ten teaspoons. For kids, this is a serious problem—drinking soda instead of milk leads to tooth problems as well as osteoporosis down the line. Not to mention, it contributes to that Toxic Belly Fat.

I'm a realist. In the transition to becoming Nutritionally Fit to Live, you may want to drink diet sodas, especially if you're stopping the full-sugar kinds. If they're decaf, even better. (And women, minimize or eliminate colas of any sort—see the "Fascinating FAToid" on page 81.) But no more than two a day—you're drinking a science-fair project in a can.

Also know this: For some people, drinking artificially sweetened beverages causes them to eat more. So try a little experiment. One day, drink only water—get some lemons, limes, oranges, or cucumbers, cut them up, and put them in a pitcher of water. Yum! Then monitor what you eat. The next day, drink your two diet sodas and monitor what you eat. If the diet sodas don't cause you to eat more, then I say okay. If they do, it's a wake-up call

Fascinating FAToid
Flushing Money Down the Drain

Americans spend a total of $40 billion on supplements, herbs, and megavitamins. Recently, a number of them have been found to be ineffective, including saw palmetto for enlarged prostate, and echinacea for colds and flu. Others, like the retinol form of vitamin A, have been found to be downright dangerous. **Bottom line:** Be sure you stay updated on the latest nutrition research. Just log onto www.drpeeke.com, and we'll keep you on top of the news you can use.

to put them on your no-go-there list. You can also experiment with drinks made with stevia, a noncaloric herb that is a natural sweetener, or bottled fructose. Both are available online or in health food stores.

Just a little juice. Looking to increase your fruit intake with juice? Nothing wrong with that. But fresh is best, and avoid the pulp-free stuff—you need that fiber.

Enjoy a cup or two of coffee. What about coffee? It may ward off Parkinson's and help counteract the effects of alcohol on the liver. Just be aware whether the caffeine is affecting your ability to sleep. And if you're pregnant, limit your intake or avoid it altogether.

Take more tea. Tea, especially green tea, has been found to have antioxidants, those great cancer-fighting properties. It has half the caffeine of coffee, and the herbal varieties have none. Five cups of green tea a day has been found to cut stroke and death from cardiovascular disease, especially in women. (With both tea and coffee, watch the sugar and cream intake.)

Alcohol in measure. As far as alcohol goes, if you have the addiction gene, stay away! For others, one drink for women, two for men may help protect your heart. Red wine in particular has been shown to have heart benefits because of our friends the antioxidants, and a new study just found that it contains melatonin, the sleep hormone. The newest research shows that in rats the red wine derivative resveratrol seems to help protect against high-fat diets as well as diabetes. A drink, by the way, is defined as one 12-ounce beer, one 6-ounce glass of wine, or 1 ounce of hard liquor. More than that, and you're increasing the

SEVERAL REASONS TO TAKE FISH OIL

Omega-3s protect against heart disease (working even better than most medicines in improving HDL cholesterol, say researchers) and inflammatory diseases such as arthritis. They help protect eyesight, improve brain function, and reduce Alzheimer's risk. Some nutritionists believe that the rise in depression is directly related to the fact that most of us are getting only one-fifth of the omega-3s we need. And a fascinating computer model study found that a diet rich in omega-3s would prevent eight times more deaths than installing defibrillators (the machines that stimulate the heart in case of a heart attack) in public buildings or inside the body.

> ## ONE MORE REASON TO TAKE FISH OIL
>
> Takers of omega-3 fish oil who also walked or ran 45 minutes three times a week for 12 weeks lost an average of 4½ pounds including Toxic Belly Fat, while those who took sunflower oil and exercised lost no weight. Neither did those who took fish oil or sunflower oil but did no exercise. The fish oil–exercise combo is a winner.

risk of liver and heart troubles, as well as other physical, emotional, and social troubles. Women need to be particularly careful. Alcohol stays in our bloodstream longer, particularly as we age, and can increase breast cancer risk. You can get some of the same heart-healthy benefits from grape juice with none of the detrimental side effects.

⇨Fit to Live Essentials⇦

Using your score from the "Are You Nutritionally Fit to Live?" test, you'll continue to build your individual program with the tips below. As in previous chapters, you'll begin according to your current level. If you're at the Survive level, focus on the first section and really master these baseline skills before moving on. If you're at the Enjoy or Challenge levels, feel free to scan the first section(s) to see if there's something you might need a refresher on; otherwise, move to your section, try those tips out, and appreciate what life is like beyond survival mode! To keep yourself on track, check out Appendix 2 for a template that will help you organize your individual plan.

TO SURVIVE:

If you received a score of 0 to 6 on the test, focus your energy here first. Once you've mastered these, feel free to move up to the tips in "To Enjoy."

1. Eat the Right Balance of Fit Carbs, Fit Protein, and Fit Fats, and Take That Multivitamin

Eat 20 to 30 percent protein, 20 to 30 percent fat, and 40 to 60 percent carbs as described in Principle #1. See "The Fit to Live Mouth Plan at a Glance" on page 118 and the week's worth of sample meals in Appendix 3 to help you get a feel for those proportions.

Fascinating FAToid

Ladies: Special Cola and Diet Cola Alert

Drinking colas, whether the diet ones or sugary, is bad for your bones. Drinking even one of these babies daily is associated with an average of 4 percent lower bone density—regardless of age, calcium and vitamin D intake, smoking, or drinking alcohol. Experts are not sure why but guess that because colas are highly acidic, calcium is leached from the bones to counteract the acid. The bottles of cola are bad for your bones.

For all of you who don't have time to keep running to a Whole Foods to pick up fresh vegetables, how do you keep this simple? Frozen. Science has clearly shown that frozen fruits and vegetables have precisely the same number of micronutrients as the fresh stuff. Just keep a boatload of frozen fruits and veggies around, so no matter what's going on, you'll be supplied. And don't forget your multivitamin!

2. When Shopping, Follow the Rule of Five, and When Eating, Follow the Rule of Two

Have large quantities of at least five different colors of fruits and veggies in your shopping cart and no more than five boxes of packaged foods. Then, in any given day, limit yourself to two processed foods. If you eat frozen white waffles for breakfast and a Hot Pocket for lunch, you're done with processed foods for the day.

VITAMIN D: NOT JUST FROM MILK ANYMORE

A lot of new research shows that vitamin D not only helps with the absorption of calcium but can help prevent ovarian and breast cancer in women, colon and pancreatic cancer in men and women, multiple sclerosis, type 1 diabetes, heart disease, seasonal affective disorder, autoimmune diseases, osteoporosis, and perhaps prostate cancer in men. We used to get this vitamin from our skin's reaction to sunlight, but we spend too much time inside now, and sunscreen blocks the reaction. Don't forget your D.

3. Steam, Grill, or Eat It Raw

When you can, steam your veggies. That way, you maintain the highest integrity of all the micro- and macronutrients. Steamers cost 10 bucks or less. Whether steaming or boiling, save the water and freeze it for a convenient stock for soup—it's loaded with nutrients. To mix things up when you grill chicken, fish, and meat, try spices and rubs rather than heavy sauces or cheese.

4. When Eating Out, Put Your A^2 to Work and Fight to Eat Right

Let's say you're going into a restaurant and nothing on the menu looks healthy. They have buttered vegetables and highly sauced chicken. (Welcome to the South.) A^2 it. Ask for the chicken with the sauce on the side. Say, "I would like the vegetables without butter." Say you're allergic to butter and you'll bust out into huge hives, and then they'll have to call 911. Make it up as you go along. Extra points for humor and creativity. As in all things, the more polite and friendly you are, the easier it is to get what you want.

5. Find a Few Healthy Choices and Stick with Them

The USDA has found that most people just keep rotating around the same seven entrées for dinners. Researchers with the National Weight Control Registry, which tracks "successful losers" who've dropped lots of weight and kept it off for years, note that people with this habit tend to keep their eating quite simple. They find a great template that works for them, and they stick with it.

Fascinating FAToid
Watch Your Caffeine Intake

Too much caffeine can make you sick. Symptoms include insomnia, tremors, sweating, nausea, diarrhea, chest pains, and heart palpitations. Caffeine poisoning often happens when you drink caffeinated beverages and take a diet supplement on top of a medicine that includes caffeine. **Bottom line:** Be aware of how much caffeine you're getting from all sources.

Fascinating FAToid

Try Tea for Waist Trimming

Tea, whether black or green, contains substances that are known appetite suppressants, diuretics, and central nervous system and muscular stimulants. **Bottom line:** Drinking tea regularly has been shown to lead to an 8-pound weight removal over a year. Here's a free bonus: Drink it iced, and you shed about another 5 pounds in a year.

To remove that Toxic Belly Fat and bank those Body Dollars, follow their practical example. To get started, you'll find a week's worth of menus in Appendix 3 for omnivores and vegetarians.

TO ENJOY:

If you scored a 7 to 13 on the test, just take a quick look at the "To Survive" suggestions. If you feel you have them covered, you can start here.

1. Go Ethnic

You've got the healthy eating template down, so now's the time to experiment. This is great for trimming Toxic Belly Fat because so many of these options are loaded with fresh whole vegetables, healthy fats, and multigrains and are low in processed foods and trans fats. Try cooking a cuisine you've never had before: Indian, Nepalese, Ethiopian, or Mediterranean. Have some fun as you give your taste buds more of a workout. Recipesource.com is a great place to get started. It lists recipes by ethnic region.

2. Expand Your Fruit and Veggie Repertoire

Ever eat a chayote? Quinoa? Dandelion greens? Pluots? Tame that Toxic Belly Fat by incorporating a wide variety of new vegetables and fruits. They fill you up, energize you throughout the day, and leave you with

> "We dare not trust our wit for making our house pleasant to our friend, so we buy ice cream."
>
> —*Ralph Waldo Emerson*

little reason to hit the vending machines. Be adventuresome at your local store and buy some of those things you've always passed by before. There are literally hundreds of vegetables and fruits. How many do you normally buy? Mix it up a bit!

3. Supplement Your Supplements

At this level of Fit to Live eating, you're taking a daily multivitamin. Now it's time to expand. If you're 40 or older, start taking omega-3s as recommended in the chart on pages 76 and 77. You'll be decreasing your risk of heart disease, as well as possibly staving off Alzheimer's disease. (And, of course, always work with your health-care practitioner as you expand your supplements.) Taking the omega-3s along with your regular physical activity is a core tool for reining in Toxic Belly Fat and staying heart healthy.

TO CHALLENGE:

If you scored a 14 to 20 on the test, just take a quick look at the "To Survive" and "To Enjoy" tips. If you feel you have them covered, you can start here.

1. Grow Your Own

Want to make sure those veggies are truly organic? Grow them yourself. The exercise you get is an added bonus. Start with easy things—green beans, tomatoes, zucchini, herbs like basil and oregano. Then challenge yourself with harder stuff—onions, asparagus, eggplant. There's an added bonus here. You'll learn patience—the same patience you need to shed Toxic Belly Fat. But the great news is that Toxic Belly Fat disappears as you toil away in the garden growing your own food. Eating these plant-based whole foods keeps that weight off for a lifetime.

Fascinating FAToid

Don't Be Tempted at the Store

Seventy percent of grocery shoppers make a list. So far, so good. But only 10 percent stick with it. Bad. Because it's the impulse purchases that tend to be the high-sugar, high-fat stuff that's causing your waistline to balloon. **Bottom line:** Stick with the list!

BE LABEL SMART

✓ Fats: When you look at fat grams, pay attention to the saturated fats and trans fats. If it has trans fats, put it back. The saturated fats number should be between 1 and 2 grams a serving. Limit grams of total fat to no more than 3 per serving and up to 5 on occasion.

✓ Sugar: Avoid products with words ending in "-ose." These are all varieties of sugar, which can add up to a lot of empty calories that the body may convert into and store as fat.

✓ Fiber: Ignore claims on the front of the box. To be a truly high-fiber food, it should have 4 grams or more per serving.

2. Take a Walk on the Wild Side

What the heck's a "neatball"? Why, it's the vegetarian answer to meatballs, of course! Ever thought of going vegetarian? Millions of people have. So long as you're making certain to watch your quality and quantity of fats, you will find that vegetarians can prevent and reverse Toxic Belly Fat. It's the whole foods—fruits, veggies, and grains—that form the fat-trimming nutritional foundation. You'll also learn that there are lots of hybrids out there like flexetarians. This means people who are vegetarian most of the time but still eat poultry and/or fish occasionally. Research has clearly shown that vegetable-laden diets are cardio protective. Try going vegetarian or flexetarian for a month and see how you feel. To get started, go to www.vrg.org/journal to find all kinds of recipes and articles about making the switch.

CHAPTER 5

Quantity: Scaling Mt. Pasta

"My doctor told me to stop having intimate dinners for four.
Unless there are three other people."
—ORSON WELLES

We eat too much. If you want to become Fit to Live, you need to get your eating under better control. How can you run to save your life if you're wearing Toxic Belly Fat from out-of-control portions? If you want to be lean, strong, and fearless, you need to maintain a better balance between what's going in and what's getting burned. It doesn't help if you know what foods to eat if you then go and eat mountains of them.

You'll be shocked at how much Portion Distortion we're suffering from. No matter what you eat, if you don't burn off the calories, the excess is stored as fat. In this chapter, you'll learn how much is appropriate and how to redefine what food "value" is so that you stop digging your grave with a knife and fork, as Governor Mike Huckabee likes to say. Controlling portions is key to Cutting Toxic Belly Fat and fueling a mind and body that can save a life—yours!

⇒Our Toxic Lifestyle⇐
Living to Eat

"Poor, darling fellow—he died of food. He was killed by the dinner table."
—DIANA VREELAND

First, there was never enough food. Famines would sweep through continents, leaving starvation and death in their wake. Even during times of plenty, however, food had great value because it took so long to access. As a hunter/gatherer and eventual farmer, we hunted, cooked, and fired it up for dinner. This was work. No time for Toxic Bellies.

We're not only hardwired for taste, but also for the *quantity* of food we need to survive. Since we come from food scarcity, we're hardwired to score food whenever we can as a preemptive strike for any upcoming famines. If we eat just enough to stay in balance and do so on a regular schedule every day, we don't turn on the "eat everything that's not tacked down" red alert in our body. It's when our Toxic Lifestyle makes our schedules chaotic that we confuse the heck out of our hardwiring. You skip a meal and then you wonder why you just ate Mt. Pasta instead of the cup of pasta you intended to eat.

We have a lot of encouragement to chow down. As the ability to produce food increased, so did the food marketing industry, whose job it is to get us to consume more. The food marketing system currently spends $36 billion a year, more than any other industry's advertising budget except carmakers. Portion Distortion has become so extreme in the

Fascinating FAToid
Forget Seconds: It's Those Firsts That Are Killing Us

People eat more if they are served large *first* portions, rather than being given small amounts and allowed to serve themselves seconds. For instance, people who were given giant popcorn buckets ate 40 to 50 percent more than those who were given smaller buckets, even when it tasted bad! When served 14-day-old popcorn, people still ate 34 percent more if it was served in a large container. **Bottom line:** Grab a smaller plate and run from large bags, boxes, and buckets!

past few decades that children, teenagers, and young adults may *never* have seen a normal portion of food in their lifetimes. Consider this:

○ Portion size for meats, starches, and dessert items has quadrupled in the past 20 years. Quadrupled!

○ The USDA serving size for a cookie is half an ounce. The average cookie sold in restaurants is 700 percent larger.

○ Twenty years ago, the average cup of coffee was 8 ounces and 95 calories from milk and sugar. Today, it's 16 ounces and 350 calories. And that's just regular coffee—one Starbuck's Grande Double Chocolate Chip Frappuccino is 580 calories.

○ In 1957, the average fast-food hamburger was 1 ounce and 210 calories. Today, it's 6 ounces and 618 calories. A medium popcorn at the movies was 3 cups in the '50s; it's now 16 cups—and 900 calories.

○ In 1986, two slices of pepperoni pizza were 500 calories; today, due to supersizing, they're 850.

○ The average serving of pasta is now five times greater than the 1-cup recommended serving size.

○ Dishes at restaurants have blown up as much as 500 percent; one meal out can overshoot your entire daily calorie allotment.

As a result of all this distortion, between 1984 and 2000, there was a greater than 15 percent increase in the average daily caloric intake per person in the United States. No wonder our waists are expanding. We need to make the portion-waistline connection. Seventy-five percent of those surveyed believe the kind of food they eat is more important than the amount, and 62 percent say restaurant portions *are the same size or smaller than in the past!* We're suffering from such Portion Distortion that even dietitians, people *paid* to know this stuff, underestimated a 1,550-calorie restaurant meal by 685 calories. That means they weren't slightly off, but miscalculated by 44 percent.

Portion Distortion is fed by packaging. Everything comes in family-size boxes with ridiculous labels that say "one serving is 6.8 grams." How much is *that*? Fast-food restaurants lure us into eating more than we'd intended to with their "value meals." We don't want to miss out on a bargain, so we buy—and consume—it all.

Watch out when you enter a restaurant. Many of us are consuming one-third of our daily calories outside our homes, and people who eat out more weigh more. Check out the calorie damage you can do at your local restaurant:

- Patty melt and fries: 1,620
- Chef salad: 930
- Chicken fajitas: 840
- Plain bagel: 500
- Spaghetti and meatballs: 1,025
- A slice of cheesecake: 640
- 32-ounce cola (plus one refill): 800

> "To lengthen thy life,
> lessen thy meals."
> —*Benjamin Franklin*

We're eating too much at home too. Dinner plates used to measure 7 to 9 inches; now the average is 11 to 13. Bigger plates make us eat more. Even the size of our silverware affects how much we eat. When given bigger spoons, people ate more ice cream. And just like other mammals, if we eat more for a while, like over holidays or on vacation splurges, when we go back to our "normal" diet, we *still* eat more than we did before. Bottom-line result of all this overeating? The average calorie consumption per person per day is now 2,757, which is 530 calories more than in 1970 and at least 300 more than even the largest man needs.

⇒Fit to Live⇐
Have a Slice—Not the Whole Cake

"Our lives are not in the laps of the gods, but in the laps of our cooks."
—LIN YUTANG

If you want to become Fit to Live to survive and Cut Your Toxic Belly Fat, you need to pay attention and get assertive. Don't just eat what's placed in front of you. Wake up, smell the huge portions, and fight for your right to appropriate amounts of food.

THE FIVE FIT TO LIVE PORTION PRINCIPLES

1. Know Your Body Dollar Budget

There are three categories of the Body Dollar budget. The first is for those people who are already at a healthy weight and want to stay there. The second is for those who carry excess weight and need to remove fat to attain a healthier weight. And the final is the small category of people who need to add weight to become healthier. We're going to concentrate on those who need to shed pounds. Let's start by figuring out where you are and what your goal should be.

A. Have a look at the "Healthy Weight Ranges" chart and become familiar with the weight ranges for your height and age. This is good to know, because it does change somewhat as you age.

HEALTHY WEIGHT RANGES

HEIGHT	WEIGHT (LB)	WEIGHT (LB)
	Ages 19–34	**Ages 35 and up**
5'0"	97–128	108–138
5'1"	101–132	111–143
5'2"	104–137	115–148
5'3"	107–141	119–152
5'4"	111–146	122–157
5'5"	114–150	126–162
5'6"	118–155	130–167
5'7"	121–160	134–172
5'8"	125–164	138–178
5'9"	129–169	142–183
5'10"	132–174	146–188
5'11"	136–179	151–194
6'0"	140–184	155–199
6'1"	144–189	159–205
6'2"	148–195	164–210
6'3"	152–200	168–216
6'4"	156–205	173–222
6'5"	160–211	177–228
Source: US Department of Agriculture and US Department of Health and Human Services		

B. Now, take the average of the range for your height and age from the "Healthy Weight Ranges" chart and use this as your ideal weight. Then, multiply your current weight by the correct Resting Calorie Requirement Factor below:

IF YOU'RE . . .	MULTIPLY BY . . .
10–30 pounds overweight	10
31–50 pounds overweight	9
51 or more pounds overweight	8

Your weight × Resting Calorie Requirement Factor = _____
This is the number of calories it takes to maintain your current weight at rest.

C. Now we need to know the whole picture. How many calories does it take to maintain your current weight taking into consideration your current level of physical activity? Multiply your total from B by the appropriate Daily Activity Factor below. Most people overestimate their physical activity, so err on the side of the smaller number.

DAILY ACTIVITY FACTOR:

1.2   very little physical activity (mostly sitting, standing, in car, lying down; most Americans are here or in the next category)
1.3   some light activity (simple housecleaning, mild to moderate walking)
1.5   moderate activities (brisk walking, biking, swimming)
2.0   heavy activities (construction work, heavy lifting, sports, athletics, runners)
2.4   highest level of athleticism (Olympian, triathlete)

Total number of calories needed at rest × Daily Activity Factor = total calories needed to maintain current weight.

But you want to remove weight, not maintain it. So, you need to strive for a daily calorie deficit. Men and women can shed up to 2 pounds of fat per week. Because there are 3,500 calories per pound, in order to shed 1 pound per week, you need to end up with a 500-calorie deficit at the end of each day for 1 week. The best way: increase your physical activity by 250 calories per day (walking 2.5 miles) while also eating 250 calories less per day. This way, you don't have to take all the calories away from your diet. You share the responsibility between what goes in (eating) and what goes out (physical activity).

2. Know the "Cost" of Certain Foods

Become aware of high-ticket items (such as butter, cheese, pizza locked and loaded with everything) and eat them sparingly. Then, strive to include the good-value items (lower-calorie such as whole grains, fruits, veggies, lean poultry, fish, and meat) as the mainstay of your daily eating.

Next, you need to learn serving sizes so you can accurately judge what a 1,400- or

1,800- or 2,000-calorie diet actually consists of. All I'm asking you to do is just once, sit down and look at the calorie counts on your favorite foods. Don't memorize exact numbers. Just be on the lookout for the high-ticket items and be careful. You can even run into problems with too much of what seems to be low-ticket food. I met a frustrated overweight woman who was mystified as to why she couldn't drop weight. She started her day out with oatmeal—that was the good news. She never looked at the label to figure out what a serving size was. That's the bad news. At my insistence, she measured her normal serving size and had a mind-blowing experience when she realized she was heaping over 2 cups into a large bowl every day with ⅓ cup of raisins along with a cup of berries. She was eating 150 percent of the recommended serving size—she was buried under mountains of healthy food! (You can get the exact calorie count for thousands of foods at www.thecaloriecounter. com or www.nutritiondata.com/index.html.)

Fascinating FAToid

Liquid Calories Count Too

If you eat a large quantity of solid food, you're more likely to eat less at the next meal than if you get the same number of calories in liquid form. Somehow, we don't register that we've overconsumed when it's a liquid. And those liquid calories really add up. Here's how you could consume a total of 3,141 calories a day without taking one bite:

8-ounce orange juice: 112

16-ounce coffee with whole milk and sugar: 350

16-ounce orange soda: 330

16-ounce Jamba juice power boost smoothie: 280

20-ounce vitamin water: 125

Venti (20 fluid ounces) Java Chip Frappuccino Blended Coffee: 720

6-ounce martini: 374

2 glasses of wine: 250

Venti (20 fluid ounces) Pumpkin Spice Creme: 600

Bottom line: Ouch! Beware your liquid calories, including those from juice places—that 16 ounces of OJ is equal to eating four oranges at once, something you are not likely to do.

The terms *portion* and *serving* are fairly interchangeable for the average person. The USDA Food Guide Pyramid (www.mypyramid.gov) has the USDA recommended servings for food groups. Any food product has a Nutrition Facts Label constructed by the food manufacturer and may or may not be in line with the USDA recommendations. Instead of relying upon these labels, which can be misleading, pick up one of those cheap little calorie-counter books—you'll see that most are based upon the USDA recommendations. Just know the general range of calories you should be sticking with and fine-tune it as changes—fat removal, altered activities—occur in your life.

3. Food Value Should Be about Quality, Not Quantity

Have you ever made a loaf of bread? I made one. I've never worked so hard in my life (this was before bread machines). That's when I discovered that food has tremendous quality value when you're the one who had to labor for it.

Being Nutritionally Fit to Live is about giving back the quality value factor to food. From now on, you will—based upon your financial ability—get the absolute best food item in every category. Say you like chocolate chip cookies. Rather than eating a whole box of cheap cookies, you'll eat one fabulous expensive cookie. By paying a lot, you'll realize that this one cookie is like a diamond. Cheap cookies are like glass chips. People who chomp on 30 cheap glass cookies *look* like it, feel like it, and live like it. People who choose the diamond look like it, feel like it, and live like it. You increase food's value by seeing things like cookies as treats rather than staples. A treat is something you have *occasionally*. That's what makes it valuable.

When I was growing up, my father would take us to the ice cream shop every Sunday. I thoroughly enjoyed it because it was a special part of our family's traditions. It was such a healthy pleasure! Then a girl named Vickie moved into our neighborhood. Vickie was overweight. One day after school, I went home with her. Usually, when I came home from school, what was waiting for me were a couple of graham crackers and sometimes an apple. At Vickie's, her mother, who was also overweight, got out ice cream and cones. I said, "You can't do that. That's a Sunday treat." Vickie looked at me proudly and said, "Ah, but in *our* family, we get it *every day*." Somehow, I knew that Vickie's mom was stripping an ice cream cone of its value, and I refused to eat it. Treasure your treats, and you'll put the value back in.

4. Savoring Is the Name of the Game

Taste research reveals that after about the second small spoon or forkful, you have optimized the entire sensual experience of something's taste. So if you are looking to really enjoy food without getting fat, it's all about savoring tiny tastes.

No one does this better than a certain A-list actress. I was invited to speak at a conference in Maui. She was there to shoot the cover of *Elle* and invited me to dinner. I watched how much she ate, remembering that in the morning, she was going to be photographed in bathing suits. I noticed that she ate an appropriate amount of greens and protein. Then the waiter came up with the dessert menu. She looked at the waiter and said, "I understand that you have fantastic desserts."

He replied, "Why, yes," and proceeded to reel off three high-calorie items.

"I'll have one of each," she said.

I thought, "Oh dear. She's a bulimic."

The desserts arrived. She took one little taste of the first item, absolutely savoring it. She did the same thing with the second dessert and the third. She paused. Then she looked around. She seemed a bit annoyed. Finally, she picked up a salt shaker and sprinkled salt over every remaining morsel.

Fascinated, I asked her what was going on. She said that her personal assistant always works it out that the minute she has her taste, the waiter takes the rest away immediately. Our waiter had apparently forgotten. I asked her, "Tell me how you figured this out."

"'I make good money and travel all over the world," she replied. "I have the opportunity to go to amazing restaurants. I'll be damned if I'm not going to *taste* each restaurant."

What I love about her solution was not only did she find a way to enjoy fabulous food,

---

IF YOU DON'T WAKE UP HUNGRY, YOU BLEW IT THE NIGHT BEFORE

They call it break*fast* for a reason. You're breaking an overnight fast. Waking up hungry is a *beautiful* little cue that you're doing it right when it comes to portions the night before. If you don't feel hunger, then you probably ate too much and/or too close to bedtime. Take the opportunity for a nice cleansing, short fast every night.

How to Judge Serving Size

Some foods are weighed in ounces. Some are measured in spoons or cups. Others, like fruits, are based on an average size. Below are some tips to help you judge what just one serving looks like.

FOOD TYPE	STANDARD SERVING	VISUAL EQUIVALENT	CALORIES
Bread, cereal, rice, and pasta	1 slice of whole wheat bread	CD case	70
	½ cup of cooked cereal, pasta, or rice	1 cupcake or ½ tennis ball	110
	1 cup dry cereal	Baseball	100–200
	1 small bagel	Hockey puck	120
	1 oz pretzels	1 cupped hand	110
Fruits and vegetables	1 medium apple/orange	Tennis ball	60–80
	1 cup chopped fruit	Fist	60–80
	¼ cup raisins	½ cupped hand	110
	1 cup vegetables (raw/cooked)	1 cupped hand	25–40
	1 medium potato	Computer mouse	160
Meat, poultry, fish, dry beans, eggs, and nuts	3 oz chicken, pork, or beef	Deck of cards	175–250
	4 oz finfish/shellfish	Checkbook	100–150
	½ cup cooked beans	Lightbulb	115
	1 oz nuts	20 peanuts/10 almonds	90
	1 egg	—	60–70
Fats, oils, and sweets	2 Tbsp peanut butter	Ping-pong ball	190–200
	1 Tbsp salad dressing	Thumb (tip to 1" joint)	45
	1 tsp butter or oil	Dime	45
	½ cup ice cream	½ tennis ball	160

Measurements at a Glance

SERVING SIZE	VISUAL EQUIVALENT
3 ounces	About the size and thickness of a deck of cards
1 ounce cheese	About the size of a domino
2 tablespoons	About the size of a walnut
1 tablespoon	About the size of a quarter
1 teaspoon	About the size of a penny
½ cup	About the size of an ice cream scoop
1 cup	About the size of a standard single-serving yogurt container
1 medium-size fruit	About the size of a small fist
2-inch slice of melon	About the width of three fingers

but when Plan A didn't work, she A²-d and found another way to make sure she didn't eat too much. That's what being Fit to Live is all about.

5. Medicate with Protein and Movement, Not Refined Fats, Sugar, or Carbs

I can't talk about portions without mentioning addictions. It's estimated that 1 in 10 Americans suffer from binge-eating disorder, a compulsion to eat even though they are full. Binge eating is 100 percent associated with depression. If you are a binge eater, please get the help you need—a team approach to your unhealthy lifestyle issues that includes antidepressant medication and therapy.

It's also *extremely* important to understand that science has now clearly shown that there is a genetic connection between sugar addiction and alcoholism. A significant number of people who have had obesity surgery are also recovering alcoholics. They shifted their addiction from alcohol to sugar and by doing so, ate enormous amounts of food. Stay as far away from refined sugars as you can if alcoholism runs in your family. Or if you are a problem drinker, please get help to become sober without resorting to mass quantities of sugar.

What about cigarette smoking, drug addiction, or other addictions? The science shows that any person who is addictive tends to have a problem experiencing the sensual feeling of satisfaction. A nonaddictive person can look at a beautiful sunset and thoroughly enjoy it. An addictive person looks at the same sunset and doesn't feel like it's enough. That's why, for an addictive person, it's not just one cigarette. It's two packs. It's never just one drink, it's always six. It's not just one piece of cake, it's the whole thing.

How come? The answer is very complex. One part of the puzzle has to do with the hormone dopamine, the happy, lustful neurotransmitter in the brain. When a nonaddictive individual looks at the sunset, their dopamine level goes up, and they feel wonderful.

Fascinating FAToid
Your Brain Will Thank You

Eating 30 percent less cut Alzheimer's symptoms in mice. Researchers are now going to look at people to see if 10 to 15 percent reductions will help with brain function. **Bottom line:** Here's another powerful mind-body reason not to overeat.

Voice of Success: "I Was a Night Stalker."

Marlyn Glickman removed 60 pounds and has maintained it for 12 years

"I thought I was eating properly because I was eating things like fat-free cookies. A box at a time. From Dr. Peeke, I learned to have one delicious cookie. I was a night stalker— in the middle of the night, I would eat whatever leftovers I had from restaurant boxes. Now in restaurants, I cut whatever I get in half and offer it to other people or give it to homeless people. I don't take leftovers home. I've also learned to really taste my food, not gulp it down. I order the most delicious dessert, have one bite, then offer it to others or put a napkin over it. It's about portion control, not denial. Denial doesn't work. If I want something, I have a taste. Otherwise, I end up eating a bunch of other stuff and then eat what I wanted all along. I also keep track of what I eat. If I find myself putting on weight, I go back to my food journal to figure out what's going on."

We're not sure why, but people who are addictive never get that fully satisfying dopamine rush. They're constantly searching for the period at the end of the sentence.

Remember too what you learned in the stress chapter. For women, high-fat, high-sugar foods increase that other feel-good hormone, serotonin, which women don't have as much of as men do. When you eat those things, stress hormone decreases, and you get more mindless about your eating. Before you know it, you've eaten 5,000 calories.

For addictive people, protein is absolutely the name of the game. When you feel the urge to anesthetize, eat protein, because it will help give you that sense of fullness and fulfillment without the empty calories. Most protein comes with some fat (low-fat string cheese), and both together are satisfying. The other thing you can do is substitute the beta-endorphins you get from moving for the missing dopamine and serotonin. Beta-endorphins are the body's own opium. That's why, when I find out someone's addictive, I become a pusher. I push physical activity.

⇒Fit to Live Essentials⇐

Using your score from the "Are You Nutritionally Fit to Live?" test, you'll continue to build your individual program with the tips below.

TO SURVIVE:

If you received a score of 0 to 6 on the test, focus your energy here first. Once you've mastered these, feel free to move up to the tips in "To Enjoy."

1. Decide What Kind of Vehicle You Are

Close your eyes for a second. Are you a four-door sedan? A little sports car? An 18-wheeler? Arnold Schwarzenegger and Venus and Serena Williams are 18-wheelers. Because of their level of muscularity, they get to eat at the 18-wheeler level. Choose the vehicle you are and start eating like it. If you're a little sports car, eat like a sports car, because you have a smaller tank than those 18-wheelers.

Here's how it can work. One day, a woman came into my office who was 5 feet 2 inches and weighed 210 pounds. I gave her the vehicle analogy. She said, "Wow! This makes sense. I'm not an 18-wheeler—I'm a little sports car—a Miata!" That became her portion credo. It kept her mindful. She cut out pictures of Miatas and pasted them on her refrigerator door and food cabinets.

Months later, she came in, and she had achieved her goal. She looked fantastic. She said, "Come outside!" There was a brand-new red Miata. "Here's the joke," she explained. "After you told me that analogy, I went to a Miata dealership and was too fat to fit in the car. I knew then that I had to change. Look at me now! I fit into my own life—and car!" With that, she popped into the driver's seat, strapped in, and drove away.

2. Use Your Power Why

Go back to what you learned in Chapter 2 about your Power Why motivation. Then when you have the choice to overeat or not, you'll say "Do I want that size 12 or 20?" Choosing your portion size carefully means you're choosing size 12. Remember that you'll look, feel,

Fascinating FAToid
The True Cost of TV Dinners

Science has shown that when people eat in front of the tube, they eat upward of two to three times the number of calories they would have eaten if they weren't in front of the TV. **Bottom line:** Like refined sugar, use the tube sparingly.

and live like the choice you just made. Keep reminding yourself of your Power Why. If it's not strong enough to help you live through the temptation, then you need to go deeper. Maybe you're really moved by a picture of your kids. It'll remind you that every choice you make impacts on them. They want you around. So do you. Act like it. Choose the right quantity, and your choice will be the life you deserve—the Fit to Live life.

3. Rest When You're Tired, Eat When You're Hungry

People often tell me, "Dr. Peeke, I'm so tired because I don't get enough sleep, so that by 3 o'clock, I eat!" Now think about this—you're tired, so you eat. Food doesn't have anything to do with sleep, people. We looked at the importance of sleep in Chapter 3. What's important here is that you don't confuse exhaustion with hunger. Otherwise, you end up eating too much of stuff that's not good for you in an attempt to boost your energy.

Pay attention to your body. Ask yourself, "Am I tired? Or am I truly hungry?" Now, if you're really hungry, then please eat responsibly. You'll learn what to snack on in Chapter 6. If you're tired, close your eyes for 5 minutes. Or—for the postgraduate crowd—meditate. But let's say you can't take a nap. You're a congressman's assistant, and he's about ready to go into the National Press Club. Get up and move around a little bit. You'll stimulate norepinephrine, an awakening hormone that will keep you going a bit longer.

4. Eat on Small Dishes and Drink a Noncaloric Beverage with Every Meal and Snack

You read earlier that we have a tendency to eat all we're given. So give yourself less by serving your food on smaller plates, cups, and bowls. Women who were given meals that were 25 percent smaller consumed 231 fewer calories and didn't feel hungry. The smaller-dishes thing is a really easy way to keep portions in line. So is the liquid trick. Liquids fill you up, and if you make yours something without calories, it can help you to not eat as much food. Again, water is best followed by herbal or green teas.

5. When in Doubt, Simply Look at What's in Front of You and Eat Half of It

Let's just say you're somewhere where you have little control over the menu (those awful business dinners with one entrée choice, or at your mom's, and she is not flexible). No worries. Eat half of whatever is in front of you. A^2 it, say to yourself, "Just because it's there doesn't mean I

> "Make hunger thy
> sauce, as a medicine
> for health."
> —*Thomas Tusser*

have to eat it. End of story." Serve yourself and start small. When served by others, divide the food in half, and wrap the rest up in advance or put it on another plate. Or split plates with someone. Work it, folks. That's the fighting Fit to Live attitude.

TO ENJOY:

If you scored a 7 to 13 on the test, just take a quick look at the "To Survive" suggestions. If you feel you have them covered, you can start here.

1. Savor and Be Mind*FULL*

No, you don't have to live in a monastery. All you have to do is pay a bit more attention. Rather than eating in front of the TV, look at what's in front of you. Divvy it up into small hills instead of a mountain. Then slow it down and really experience the flavors and textures. When people eat slower, they eat less. People who are mind*FULL* enjoy what they're eating more, and feel full much faster. People who are mind*LESS* don't. When you savor, you save the calories.

2. Try the 80 Percent Rule

Remember that old tip about stopping before you're completely full because it takes 20 minutes to know if you're full? That's why I teach people the 80 percent rule—stop when you're 80 percent full so that when your brain catches up with your stomach, you haven't eaten too much. The sense of fullness is created by a number of factors. When you stop at 80 percent, you'll feel satisfied 20 minutes later, instead of bloated and in pain. You folks with the obesity gene (you know who you are) need to teach yourself this trick. When you carry the obesity gene, you know the feeling of starved, and you know the feeling of stuffed. But you have no idea what full feels like. It's not easy to slap on the brakes since yours don't work. That's why you have to be on red alert and consciously plan to stop.

3. Create Single-Serving Treats of Your Nonbingeables

First make a list of your bingeables. You know—those treats that once you eat one, you've eaten the whole package. Now, make a list of treats that are nonbingeables. Those are the treats that, while incredibly delicious and satisfying, do not cause you to eat more than a serving or two at a time. If chocolate is a nonbingeable, buy a bar of fabulous organic chocolate rich in flavonoids and antioxidants. Break it up into 2-ounce single servings, put each into a small snack bag, and store them in the fridge or freezer. Then when you're in the mood for a treat, you've already got the right portion.

TO CHALLENGE:

If you scored a 14 to 20 on the test, just take a quick look at the "To Survive" and "To Enjoy" tips. If you feel you have them covered, you can start here.

1. Always Leave with a Doggy Bag

Whenever you eat out, challenge yourself to bring something home (unless the food was awful). Or give it to a homeless person, like my patient Marlyn. That way, you know you aren't eating too much.

2. Take a Cruise and Actually Lose Weight

I'm kidding. This challenge is about proving to yourself that you can go on a vacation and maintain yourself. Or go up no more than 2 or 3 pounds. Then, when you return home, how quickly can you regroup and trim that Toxic Belly Fat again? People who are Nutritionally Fit to Live learn how to regroup quickly and get right back on track.

3. Parcel Out Party Portions

Show you can go to any social occasion—your best friend's birthday party, your mother's house for Thanksgiving—and not overconsume. Put your Fit to Live to Survive and Enjoy skills together and practice them at social occasions. Impress yourself with the fact that whether you're at the White House or your house, you know how to incorporate healthy treats into your Fit to Live nutrition.

CHAPTER 6

Frequency: Dashboard Dining, Anyone?

"A smiling face is half the meal."
—LATVIAN PROVERB

Let's get a quick reality check. Who remembers the last time the whole family sat down to dinner, hanging out and talking about the day? If you live alone, ever notice that you're eating mindlessly in front of the tube or newspaper, or that you simultaneously eat while you stumble around the house multitasking? When you are Nutritionally Fit to Live, you have an increased consciousness of the need to take time to sit and savor.

In this chapter, I'm going to look at when and how we're eating, and how it really should be. I know that you can't make every meal a sit-down experience. I'm a Dashboard Dining expert—my second home is an airport. You don't have to sacrifice high quality for portability.

⇒Our Toxic Lifestyle⇐
Stuff It In—Fast

"Who bothers to cook TV dinners? I suck them frozen."
—WOODY ALLEN

In the past, the Norman Rockwell vision of the family sitting around the table was not far off the mark. Not just one meal either—all three were eaten together, with Dad coming in from the fields and the kids coming home from school for the midday meal. Mom was home, making three meals a day from scratch. Eating out was a rare treat, if it happened at all. There were no such things as fast-food restaurants. As recently as 1926, a hamburger and fries ranked 19th in a list of New Yorker's top meals. Number one? Corned beef and cabbage, followed by pork loin. Both items take a long time to cook—and to eat.

Snacks were things like penny candy that tended to be sold one at a time at the old-fashioned candy counter. Snacks were so unusual that when potato chips were first invented in the 1880s, they were sold as part of restaurant meals. By suppertime, especially in the wintertime, it was dark. You ate dinner and went to sleep—no evening snacking.

In the 20th century, a number of things happened. Electricity opened up the possibility of eating much later in the evening. Women entered the workforce in huge numbers, and meal preparation, something that traditionally took all day, needed to be compressed. Time spent on meal prep and cleanup went from over 40 hours in the early 1900s to less than 10 hours by 1975 and has gotten squeezed from there. The assembly line that first brought us cars was applied to food service—enter the fast-food restaurant. And, remem-

Fascinating FAToid
Speed Up, Value Down

In the United States, some of the first dashboard lunches were pizzas. Bought in the morning by Italian factory workers in the early 20th century, they were eaten for lunch, heated up on top of radiators. **Bottom line:** Because we no longer labor physically, we end up wearing those pizzas as Toxic Belly Fat.

ber all those hours we're now working? People who have jobs barely have time to eat anymore, much less cook. We're spending 14 percent less time breaking for lunch compared with 10 years ago.

The result of all these factors is to grab food whenever and wherever we can. Walking, talking, at our computers, at the conference table: We're eating everywhere and always. We want food fast, and we want someone else to make it. Eating out is now so common that on any given day, more than 4 out of 10 adults have at least one meal at a restaurant. "Time and convenience" ranks as the number one reason we eat away from home, surpassing "variety" recently for the first time. Speed is one of the reasons we now spend more money on fast food than on new cars or computers, or all books, music, videos, and movies combined.

When we do "cook" at home, only 55 percent of dinners have even one homemade dish. Even in France, a nation known for its love of cooking, 7 in 10 shoppers now use ready-prepared meals. We're cooking so little that recipes now assume we know nothing—like greasing the pan means putting the oil on the inside, not the outside! Cooking teachers report that many people use their ovens only to store clothes.

Most of these convenience foods are of the fat-salt-calorie trifecta:

○ One-quarter of adults and one-third of kids in the United States eat fast food every day. Yes, you read right. Every day.

○ Americans now consume 100 acres of pizza a day and an average of three hamburgers and four orders of fries a week.

○ We're now eating 6.6 billion pounds of salty snacks—chips, pretzels, etc. That's 22 pounds per person per year. And there are over 100 brands of potato chips alone.

Fascinating FAToid
Use Some Girth Control, Please!

In 1970, Americans spent about $6 billion on fast food; in 2001, they spent more than $110 billion. **Bottom line:** Look at your waistline right now and realize you're wearing your fast-food junk choices.

Fascinating FAToid

Hold the Salt

A recent study found that we could save 150,000 lives a year in the United States if we cut our salt intake in half. That's because salt raises the risk of high blood pressure, heart disease, and stroke, at least in some people. But our salt intake continues to rise, mostly from processed fast foods. **Bottom line:** Fresh foods are low in salt, and it takes only a brief time—a few weeks, at most—to get used to the taste of foods with less salt.

It's not convenience that's the problem, but what the fast products are. High-fat, high-carb, high-salt, and high-sugar foods dominate the quick products we're consuming. All those cheap meals come with an added cost—an average additional 10 pounds of Toxic Belly Fat and twice the chance to develop insulin resistance, a precursor to diabetes, as compared with folks who don't patronize such places. In addition, as your fast-food dining frequency increases, your intake of vital nutrients such as vitamins A and C, calcium, phosphorus, and magnesium decreases, and your intake of dangerous trans fats increases.

Consumers say they want healthier fast foods but have trouble finding appealing choices. Part of the problem is that the junk is everywhere—in every 7-Eleven and grocery store aisle, at every airport kiosk, in every handy-dandy vending machine. When you're out and about, you have to search hard for something decent. But even when healthier choices are available, we're not making them. For instance, even with a bunch of choices available, 98 percent of McDonald's customers still don't order a salad, and the double cheeseburger is still the top seller—with all its 460 calories, 23 grams of fat, 1,140 milligrams of sodium, and whopping 1 gram of fiber.

If you want to become lean and strong, as well as stay Alert and Vertical, it's time to stop falling asleep at the meal. By now, you're well aware of the consequences on your belly and your life of continuing on this toxic high-fat, high-sugar, high-salt junk-food path. Time for a little humble acceptance: You've got to find a different way to eat on the go if you want to Cut the Toxic Belly Fat and become Fit to Live.

⇒Fit to Live⇐
Grab and Go, Done Well

"Creativity is mastery of simplicity."
—CHRISTOPHER ZEEMAN

The Fit to Live attitude accepts that we do need quick eating solutions. And we do need healthy snacks. I prefer to call them small, balanced feedings. Being Nutritionally Fit to Live is about eating appropriate foods at appropriate times.

THE FIVE FIT TO LIVE DASHBOARD DINING PRINCIPLES

1. Eat Every 3 to 4 Hours

Remember our warm-blooded mammals from Chapter 4? If there are too many hours between feeding, any warm-blooded mammal will overeat substantially, ofttimes *twice* what they would normally. Why? Because their brain and hormonal system tells them they're in famine, so they eat more to store up.

We humans don't pay attention to this primal reality. Instead, we go hours and hours without eating and then gorge on Bacchanalian feasts because we've set off our famine alert. That's why from now on, you must have some food every 3 to 4 hours. Period. You'll be in much better control of what you're eating and how much.

Babies and young children need to be fed roughly every 3 to 4 hours, right? But we become such smarty-pants when we grow up. We blow off these primal needs. Instead we say, "I can't eat. I have a very important meeting." We're not listening to our inner child.

If you eat the right amounts of the right foods, you'll experience that nice little feeling of hunger every 3 to 4 hours. That empty feeling is an alarm clock from your body that it's appropriate to have a little something. The majority of people who are doing the 24/7 eating rarely ever experience the sense of hunger. When they do, they panic and overeat immediately.

So in addition to breakfast, lunch, and dinner, have a midmorning and midafter-

> "There is a difference between eating and dining. Dining is an art."
> —*Yuan Mei*

noon healthy small feeding. The midmorning feeding is optional because you have to have had breakfast 3 hours earlier in order to require that feeding. If you finished breakfast at 9 a.m., and you'll eat lunch around noon to 1 p.m., you don't need a midmorning feeding.

The between-meal feedings are the perfect cure for overeating at lunch and dinner. You won't show up for these meals foaming at the mouth and will end up eating appropriate amounts.

SAMPLE SMALL FEEDINGS

NEED REFRIGERATOR/FREEZER	NO REFRIGERATION NEEDED
2 ounces light havarti cheese	1 cup freeze-dried strawberries, raspberries, bananas
1 fruit and yogurt smoothie bar	
1 Skinny Cow chocolate mousse bar	$\frac{1}{2}$ cup bran cereal, such as Back to Nature Hi-Fiber Multibran cereal, combined with $\frac{1}{4}$ cup raisins and $\frac{1}{4}$ cup nuts, such as pecans, almonds, walnuts, and pistachios
1 single-serve fat-free pudding or tapioca	
Large slice of watermelon	
1 all-fruit frozen ice pop	1 cup freeze-dried assorted veggies
1 light ice cream bar	1 cup carrot sticks and 4 or 5 walnuts
1 light ice cream sandwich	$\frac{1}{3}$ cup Genisoy Zesty Barbeque or Clockit soy nuts
6 ounces Breyers Light Probiotic Plus yogurt	
10 ounces Stonyfield Farm Light Smoothie drinkable yogurt	Iced diet green tea beverage
	1 cup almond milk, refrigerated after opening
6 ounces DanActive drinkable yogurt	$\frac{1}{2}$ bag light popcorn, such as Orville Reden-bacher's Smart Pop
Pete's Tofu2Go (Very Berry or Thai Tango)	
2 ounces Laughing Cow Light Gourmet Cheese Bites	Fresh fruit, such as an apple, pear, nectarine, banana, plum, or orange
	1 Luna or Extend bar
1 low-fat string cheese	Banana and 1 small handful pistachios
1 single-serve low-fat yogurt	1 serving reduced-fat peanut butter on multigrain crackers
1 single-serve low-fat cottage cheese	
	Dried apple rings
	Single-serve applesauce or apple cranberry sauce

2. The Biggest Mistake You Can Make Is to Eat Most of Your Calories at the End of the Day

There are two reasons that this is true: First, because when we eat at night, we're tired, more apt to be "asleep at the meal," and make poor choices. We tend to eat high-calorie, high-fat, high-refined-sugar junk—a box of cookies or a giant bag of chips. The calories just sit there turning into Toxic Belly Fat while we sleep. And because our metabolism slows as we age, the older you get, the more murderous this practice becomes. You have to spread the wealth of healthy whole foods throughout the day. That's why I recommend you consume 70 percent of your daily calories by the end of the midafternoon snack and finish dinner by 8 or 8:30 p.m.

If you're out at a function and have no choice but to eat later, then keep with the every 3 to 4 hours rule, and eat a small balanced feeding (yogurt with sliced almonds, a low-fat string cheese, cottage cheese, a cracker with reduced-fat peanut butter), and your hunger will be controlled. Then remember that *the later you eat, the lighter you eat.* Hit the veggies and protein.

When you're doing the 3- to 4-hour eating thing, you're less likely to come home and feast on predinner, dinner, and postdinner calories and inhale 1,000 calories that you don't need and will definitely wear the next morning. Think I'm kidding? A large handful of nuts and that martini are over 700 calories.

Voice of Success: "If I Can Do That Here, I Can Do It Anywhere."

Lisa Behnke removed 30 pounds of fat

"When I'm home, I eat well. The trouble is I'm never home. I fly every week and eat dinner out every weekday. I used to eat everything they gave me on the plane, thinking that I didn't know when my next meal would be. Now, I carry a high-protein, high-fiber power bar and dissect the meals to get the protein and veggies only. When I walk into one of my favorite restaurants, I ask myself, 'Can I find something here I like that's good for me?' Even when I 'splurge,' I order a chocolate dessert and take one bite.

"Three weeks into working with Dr. Peeke, I was leading a workshop, and they brought in Caesar salad and pizza for lunch. I had no time to go elsewhere. I noticed the salad had dressing on the side, and there was one pizza with grilled chicken. I took the chicken and greens, and squeezed on a lemon. It took 30 seconds. I thought, if I can do that here, I can do it anywhere."

Your brain can be trained to avoid evening-hour food frenzies. One way is to stay out of the kitchen after dinner. Period. Try something I learned from a patient. I asked her what time of day was worst in terms of her eating. She said, "Around 4- to 5-ish."

I looked at her and said, "Come on, 'fess up. Most red-blooded folks are foraging until they hit the sack. Then they wake up hating themselves in the morning."

"Oh no," she said. "I've never done that. My mother had five children. We would go back into the kitchen as she was cleaning up and want to forage. She had my dad make a wooden sign. One side said 'open' and the other 'closed.' If we snuck in when the kitchen was closed, our allowance was docked. I learned fast. When I got married, my mother gave me the sign. My problem is eating when the kitchen is open, not when it's closed." If evening noshing is a problem, make a sign for yourself—and follow it!

3. Eating Every 3 to 4 Hours Isn't License to Eat Mass Quantities of Junk

It's that integrated approach, remember? Follow an appropriate fit (Chapter 4) and appropriately portioned (Chapter 5) intake of food. In the best of worlds, you want to have a combination of fit protein, fit carbs, and fit fat at each 3- to 4-hour interval. That means three meals and two snacks. You should have a 3- to 4-ounce serving of protein (poultry, lean red meat, fish, 8 fluid ounces of low-fat or fat-free dairy, or larger servings of vegetarian combos) at each meal and a 1- to 2-ounce serving of protein at each snack—1.5 cups low-fat cottage cheese, low-fat string cheese, 6 to 8 ounces yogurt, 1 tablespoon reduced-fat peanut butter, 10 almonds or walnuts. Plus, unlimited nonstarchy vegetables and one serving of fruit and whole grains at each feeding. (See "The Fit to Live Mouth Plan at a Glance" on page 118.)

Don't worry about being a purist. You come home, and there's nothing else around but a bunch of frozen vegetables and some low-fat cheese. That's better than fast food. Got some Egg Beaters? Make an omelet, throw in some of the half-wilted vegetables that are sitting in the refrigerator, and you've got vegetables with protein. If you have a little bit of fat-free milk, soy milk, or protein powder, throw that into the omelet, and you get a little extra protein. A^2 and do the best you can at the time. That's what being Nutritionally Fit to Live is all about.

4. When You Grab and Go, Grab and Go Fit

When I was an intern and resident, I carried not one, but two beepers. One was just for routine admissions, and one was for codes (resuscitations). Inevitably, when I said the magic words, "Let's go to the cafeteria and have a meal," one or the other went off. That's when I discovered the wonderful world of peanut butter and jelly sandwiches. I was Fit to Live to survive as I ate them when I had no other recourse but vending machines. (Of course, it took me a while to be able to eat PB&J again after 3 years of training!)

Like me, you don't have to handgrind your own nut butters to eat healthfully. There are a whole slew of great options.

Professionally prepared foods. Whole Foods delis, which prepare and deliver food; Jenny Direct, which will deliver Jenny Craig items; Zone Chefs that will make meals-to-go based on the Zone diet; and now grocery stores can deliver foods to your door to keep you well stocked for that grab-and-go moment.

Home-prepped foods. Can't afford someone else doing it for you? Buy mixed lettuce in bulk and sliced oven-roasted chicken breasts. Cook a boatload of stuff on Sunday, like soup or grilled fish or chicken, and freeze in single-serving containers. Or buy a package of whole wheat pita and freeze it. When it's time to go, whip that baby out of the freezer. (That's the beauty of pitas. They're unbingeable. When was the last time you met anyone who ate 35 pitas?) Nuke it for about 15 seconds. Then take 2 to 3 ounces of low-fat cheese, cut it up, throw it into the pita, nuke it again for about 10 seconds. Then grab a piece of fruit, and you're on your way out. You have protein, carbs, and fat, all in a beautiful balance that you can eat in your car for easy and healthy Dashboard Dining. The entire thing takes no more than 2½ minutes to make.

Juice. I have an Omega juicer. One of my favorite juices is a mix of apples, carrots, and ginger. Whir for a couple of minutes; throw it into a thermos, and go. It's a no-brainer way to be able to enjoy the full micronutrients and macronutrients of fruits and vegetables. Make it a complete meal by adding in some milk, yogurt, or protein powder.

Meal replacement drinks. At those words, you might point your nose to the ceiling and say, "What happened to whole food?" If you're running around like the grand majority of us, a protein shake made with protein powder, whey or soy, and fresh or frozen fruit with either some water or fat-free milk will keep you rocking and rolling for 3 hours and out of the vending machine.

> "Dine, v: to eat a good dinner in good company, and eat it slow."
>
> —*Ambrose Bierce*

Energy bars. Most of these should not be used as a meal replacement unless there are *absolutely* no decent alternatives. Like you're on a plane at LaGuardia, and the captain gets on the mike and says, "Well, the good

Fascinating FAToid

Lack of Time Is No Excuse

Half of those with Toxic Belly Fat blame it on their busy lifestyle. **Bottom line:** Those who are Fit to Live accept that you've got to plan. Those who don't, wear their out-of-control lifestyle around their waistline.

news is we're going to Washington. The bad news is we're number 33 in line." Is this ideal? Of course not. But it will help you to A^2 in response to a bad situation.

Not all energy bars are created equal. Many are too high in fat. Please refer to the chart on page 114 to find some good examples of energy bars that might be right for you. Watch portion size too. One serving of 150 to 200 calories for women and up to 300 calories for a man should do the trick quite nicely.

5. Anyone for a Grape-Nuts Dinner?

No more "that's not a dinner food." Any healthy food combo works at any meal or any snack and *definitely* as you do grab-and-go. How about a two-omelet day? Chicken or fish for breakfast is perfectly fine. Think in terms of scoring fit carbs, proteins, and fats, rather than a dining category based on time of day.

⇨Fit to Live Essentials⇦

Using your score from the "Are You Nutritionally Fit to Live?" test, you'll continue to build your individual program with the tips below.

TO SURVIVE:

If you received a score of 0 to 6 on the test, focus your energy here first. Once you've mastered these, feel free to move up to the tips in "To Enjoy."

1. Whenever Possible, Sit and Savor with Butt on Chair

Carefully study your eating places. Does your kitchen look like a grenade just hit it? Are there piles of newspapers, bills, and mail thrown on your dining room table? No wonder you're not sitting when you eat. You *can't*!

Make new rules. No eating in bed. No watching the tube while you're eating. Pay attention to the preparation and the ritual of eating. How about treating yourself to sitting in a real chair with a place setting in front of you, nice music playing in the background, and lit candles? Whip out your best china. Never wait for guests.

Whenever possible, do it for small feedings, do it for meals. Notice I said "whenever possible." I know you can't do this every day. Just do it when you can. It helps remind you to steer clear of mindless eating.

2. Give Yourself Permission to Dashboard Dine

How many times have you heard that you shouldn't eat on the run? Get real. You've got to eat every 3 to 4 hours. Unless you never leave your house, that means you have to Dashboard Dine a lot. Plan to eat in the car (while you're parked, of course!). Make sure your car is loaded with napkins and plasticware. When you accept Dashboard Dining, you plan for it. If you fail to plan, you plan to fail.

3. Get Armed and Dangerous with Portable Normals

From now on, BYOF: Bring Your Own Food. That means thinking before you head out the door so you will have access to fit protein, carbs, and fats every 3 to 4 hours. Most protein requires some form of refrigeration. Do you have access to a fridge at work? Great—load it up with low-fat string cheese, yogurt, hard-cooked egg whites, cottage cheese, etc., as well as vegetables and fruit.

When there's no refrigeration, or if you're a surgeon or firefighter or police officer or other person whose work comes with mobility, you have to get more creative, especially with protein. That's where grab-and-go foods come in: healthy foods that don't require

---

SALT RED ALERT

Many time-starved folks pop frozen entrées into the microwave. Beware—these usually come with a hefty dose of salt, often 700 to 900 milligrams as a preservative. If you are an average person, you shouldn't be having more than 1,500 milligrams all day! Be sure to check out the sodium level on the label, and no matter what, don't add any more. And if you have high blood pressure, look for low-sodium products.

Fascinating FAToid

They're Making It Easier

The CEO of 7-Eleven has just mandated that franchise owners add racks of bananas, pears, apples, and sliced carrots to their stores around the world. **Bottom line:** You can find healthy options in more places every day.

refrigeration and that you can have with you at all times. (See "Sample Small Feedings" on page 107.) One of my favorite is reduced-fat crunchy peanut butter (if it's not a bingeable of yours) on some multigrain crackers. Put it into a ziptop bag, and there's your small feedings for the day. Or carry an appropriate meal replacement energy bar if there's no whole food accessible (car, train, plane, elevators on way to meeting).

Do you commute? Load the car at all times with 2-ounce ziptop bags of homemade tropical mix. Go to Trader Joe's, or Whole Foods, or anywhere they have the big vats of dried fruits and nuts, and make your own combo. Stretch out those calories with a high-fiber cereal such as Fiber One. Nuts, especially raw or dry roasted cashews, walnuts, and almonds, are fabulous; they offer fit protein, carbs, and fats in one tiny package. Never go anywhere without some. Ditto nutritious power bars. Commute by bus or carpool? Pack the stuff in your briefcase. And don't forget the water. Now you've got your emergency backup system.

4. Limit Evening Calories

In the best of all worlds, have no solid food for 2 hours prior to hitting the sack. This takes a little planning. If you go to bed at 11, you should be done eating by 9. Best would be 8, with 70 percent of your calories consumed by midafternoon. If you can't help eating late, remember this rule: *The later you eat, the lighter you eat.* Especially over age 40, whatever you overeat at night, you wear on your waist in the morning. And quite frankly, eating before you go to bed is a significant cause of stomach reflux, which, if it becomes a chronic problem, can lead to esophageal disease and even cancer. Best to hit the sack with a mostly empty stomach.

Need to wean yourself off of funky nighttime eating? Start by eating half of what you normally consume. Let's say you normally eat five cookies. Okay, eat 2½. That's the quantity issue. The *quality* issue is that cookies probably aren't the world's greatest thing at night. How about some fresh fruit with a little bit of yogurt? Are these calories after

(continued on page 116)

MEAL REPLACEMENT BARS AND DRINKS BY THE NUMBERS

ITEM	CALORIES	TOTAL FAT (GRAMS)	SAT'D FAT (GRAMS)	SODIUM (MG)	CARBS (GRAMS)	FIBER (GRAMS)	PROTEIN (GRAMS)
Bars for Endurance (High-Carb)							
Garden of Life—Summer Berry	230	3.5	1	25	47	4	3
Larabar—Pecan Pie	220	14	1	0	22	4	3
Nature's Path Organic—blueberry, flax, soy	200	3	1	125	39	7	7
Bars for Strength (High-Protein)							
Pure Protein-Chocolate Deluxe	170	4.5	3.5	140	17	2	20
Cliff Builders Cocoa-Dipped Double Decker	270	8	5	240	30	4	20
Power Bar Protein Plus	300	6	3.5	150	38	1	23
Bars That Control Blood Sugar Levels							
Extend Bar	130	3	0	150	9	5	12
Glucerna	220	7	3.3	80	32	2	10
Gender-Specific Bars							
Male:							
Met-Rx Big 100—Peanut Butter Cookie Dough	360	5	1.5	200	51	2	27
Myoplex Lite—Peanut Caramel Crisp	180	6	3	270	25	8	15
Jay Bar—Fudge Brownie	220	10	1	210	27	6	14
Female:							
Luna Sunrise Strawberries and Cream—AM Nutrition for Women	180	4	2	95	29	5	8
Luna Chai Tea—Whole Nutrition Bar for Women	180	4	3	125	27	3	10
Slim Fast Optima On-the-Go Milk Chocolate Peanut	220	5	3	160	34	3	8

ITEM	CALORIES	TOTAL FAT (GRAMS)	SAT'D FAT (GRAMS)	SODIUM (MG)	CARBS (GRAMS)	FIBER (GRAMS)	PROTEIN (GRAMS)
Soy-Based Bars							
Revival	250	9	4	250	33	4	19
South Beach Diet—Caramel Peanut Crisp	210	7	2.5	350	25	5	19
Dr. Soy Chocolate Brownie	180	4	3	150	26	1	11
Bars with Natural Ingredients							
ReBar Grains and Greens	160	1.6	not listed	21	32	5.6	4.1
Power Bar Nut Naturals	210	10	1	180	20	3	10
Odwalla Super Protein	230	4.5	1.5	160	31	4	16
Bars for Kids							
Cliff Organic Z-Bar—Chocolate Chip	130	4	1.5	100	24	3	3
High-Fiber Bars							
Renew LifeOrganic Fiber Bar—Lemon Burst	160	3.5	0	30	35	14	2
Bars That Are Really Candy							
Maya Chocolate Coffee (Dairy-Free Vegan)	190	11	1	0	25	5	4
Tigers Milk—Peanut Butter	200	10	3	125	28	1	9
Carb Solutions—Fudge Almond Brownie	230	10	4.5	220	22	2	20
Meal-Replacement Powders (2 scoops)							
Metagenics Ultra-meal—Natural Vanilla	160	2	not listed	180	24	4	15
Xymogen Insulean Whey Functional Food	170	2	1	36	18	1	21
Slimstyles Orange Cream	226	7	3	260	13	5	22

dinner? Yes. But it's a hell of a lot better than having a sleeve of cookies. Eventually you say to yourself, "I don't really need all that. Maybe I'll have an apple."

In the transition to becoming Nutritionally Fit to Live, I'm giving you a hundred calories at night for a final small feeding. A low-calorie frozen fudge bar is fine. There are plenty of options out there. Just make sure to have it 1 to 1½ hours before bed, and keep the quantity down and the quality up. And let go of it when you can.

5. Show Off Your Ability to A² and Find Healthy Food Wherever You Are

There is *no* excuse for eating junk. Think of it like the ultimate reality show: Can you score healthy food no matter where we put you? Starbucks is everywhere. They sell grilled chicken on a bed of greens as well as yogurt. Can you go into a W. H. Smith at an airport and make it work? There's water—that's good. There are some unsalted nut combinations that actually work well as long as you watch portions very closely. That trail mix is not bad so long as you really watch portions and avoid the chocolate and chocolate yogurt-coated stuff. There are healthier-option energy bars sold in most stores.

Or you're driving in the middle of nowhere, and all there is are fast-food restaurants. Show 'em watcha' got. A² it. Order a salad with everything on the side. You'll end up with a bunch of green salad, a packet of chicken, and a packet of vegetables. Throw in a few croutons or ditch them. There will also be dressing. Dressing is the killer. Twist and twizzle with your fork to get a couple teaspoons at most, and throw the rest away.

TO ENJOY:

If you scored a 7 to 13 on the test, just take a quick look at the "To Survive" suggestions. If you feel you have them covered, you can start here.

Fascinating FAToid
The Benefits of Family Dinner

Eating together as a family creates happier marriages, teenagers' healthier sense of identity and academic achievement, and stronger family ties. Children and teens who eat at the dinner table are thinner, fitter, and healthier than kids who don't. **Bottom line:** We're not talking forever here—20 minutes together is all it takes.

Fascinating FAToid

Avoid the Vending Machine and Minibar Pounds

The average person buys food or beverages from a vending machine 1.52 times a day. Those who do it the most—almost three times a day—also eat out the most often and are more likely to be obese. Minibars are similarly dangerous for travelers. **Bottom line:** Pack your own snacks so you won't be tempted. And say no when the hotel clerk is about to hand you the minibar key.

1. B.Y.O.F.F.

Bring your own fun food. That means instead of boring yourself to tears with the feedings you learned to use while practicing how to be Fit to Live to survive, get creative. How about snackin' on edamame (soybeans in pods)? What about carrots dipped in hummus? Check out "Sample Small Feedings" on page 107 for more options.

2. Instead of Hit and Run, Drive and Enjoy

If you're going to Dashboard Dine, do it in style. Spend some bucks and get a fabulous thermos and reusable containers with matching lids. Tupperware and other brands now offer the adult version of the lunch box. Outfit yourself with gear that you like and enjoy using.

3. Eat 'n' Walk

Closely pair snacking with moving. Eat your midmorning and midafternoon small feedings before or after a walk. Or, if you've just finished eating in the car, get out and move around a bit before heading into the meeting. When you combine your feedings with movement, you keep your energy balance equation—calories in and out—in better balance and reduce the chances of seeing that food around your middle.

TO CHALLENGE:

If you scored a 14 to 20 on the test, just take a quick look at the "To Survive" and "To Enjoy" tips. If you feel you have them covered, you can start here.

1. Plan for a Long-Haul Challenge

Going to take a long drive, say 8 to 10 hours? Can you arrive at your destination having been armed and dangerous with enough healthy snacks and meals to have avoided

> "We should look for someone to eat and drink with before looking for something to eat and drink, for dining alone is leading the life of a lion or wolf."
>
> —*Epicurus*

"fast-food regret"? How about that coast-to-coast plane trip, or hoppin' onboard for that European or Asian vacation or business trip? It's all about planning. Bring some portable feedings along with you, and say "no thanks" to the science-fair projects you're offered on most airline flights. These portable feedings are also a godsend when you're stuck in a foreign airport waiting for a connection and you don't have the currency to buy some food.

2. Survive the Stress-Out

Go to the big-time stress place. You've got a deadline, you're giving a talk the next day, you're talking to the boss about a promotion. Times of high stress are where those head-in-the-fridge binges tend to happen. Meet the challenge by having a plan of action to neutralize the tendency to stick something in your mouth. Most animals under stress get really oral—cats chew your carpet, dogs chew grass, and you chew anything that's not tacked down. You've got the skills. You can do this. Chew gum and put everything you've learned in this book into gear.

THE FIT TO LIVE MOUTH PLAN AT A GLANCE

<----------------70 percent of calories consumed---------------->   8 p.m. (stop eating)

BREAKFAST	A.M. SMALL FEEDING	LUNCH	P.M. SMALL FEEDING	DINNER	100-CALORIE TREAT
Unlimited nonstarchy veggies	Unlimited nonstarchy veggies	Unlimited nonstarchy veggies	Unlimited nonstarchy veggies	Unlimited nonstarchy veggies	Low-fat (0–2g), low-sugar (10–20g) treat
3 to 4 oz fit protein	1 to 2 oz fit protein	3 to 4 oz fit protein	1 to 2 oz fit protein	3 to 4 oz fit protein	
1 fit carb serving (fruit or whole grain)	1 fit carb serving (fruit or whole grain)	1 fit carb serving (fruit or whole grain)	1 fit carb serving (fruit or whole grain)	1 fit carb serving (fruit or whole grain)	

SERVING SIZES AND SUGGESTIONS

UNLIMITED NONSTARCHY VEGETABLES	3 TO 4 OZ FIT PROTEIN	1 TO 2 OZ FIT PROTEIN	FIT CARBS	FIT FATS	100-CALORIE TREATS
Broccoli	Palm-size chicken breast	1¼ cups cottage cheese	1 slice whole wheat bread	10 almonds	1 fudgsicle
Asparagus	Palm-size turkey breast	2 oz soy cheese	½ cup steamed brown rice	¼ avocado	1 Tbsp almond butter on celery
Carrots	Wild salmon	⅓ cup soy nuts	½ cup whole grain pasta	20 peanuts	½ small whole wheat pita and 3 Tbsp hummus
Green pepper	Veggie burger	1 cup low-fat yogurt	½ cup barley	1 Tbsp olive oil	Low-fat pudding
Spinach	Tuna	2 oz tofu	½ whole wheat bagel	12 walnut halves	1 Tbsp low-fat peanut butter on whole wheat crackers
Tomato	Lean beef	1 low-fat string cheese	1 whole wheat wrap	1 Tbsp canola oil	1 square organic chocolate
Zucchini	Lean pork	2 oz low-fat cheese	½ cup oatmeal	1 Tbsp safflower oil	4 oz protein smoothie

CHAPTER 7

Stop Dieting and Start Shedding Fat

"I've been on a constant diet for the past 2 decades. I've lost a total of 789 pounds. By all accounts, I should be hanging from a charm bracelet."
—ERMA BOMBECK

I f you want to cut your excess Body Fat off permanently, you'll have to swear off fad diets from now on. Raise your right hand and repeat after me: "I _____(your name) am making a commitment to myself to run in the opposite direction when another fad diet hits the bookstores, and instead embrace my Fit to Live sustainable, life-long nutrition plan."

In this chapter, I'm going to show you that there are many healthy eating options out there. There will never ever be one that works for everyone. They all work, if you pick and choose from them, like bellying up to a buffet table of choices. What I'm going to do is to give you some guiding principles to help you steer clear of the fads and concentrate on a healthy mindset that will augment any of the healthy eating plans you want to use.

⇒Our Toxic Lifestyle⇐
Mountains of Delicious Food Calling Your Name

"[The low-carb food industry] was aimed squarely at the age-old pursuit of getting thin while eating whatever you want, which, of course, never works."
—*THE WASHINGTON POST*, 2005

As we've seen, throughout most of human history, dieting was a moot point because we struggled to get enough food. When food became abundant and we began to move less, not only did our waistlines explode but so did the diet industry with its endless procession of diet fads: the grapefruit diet, the low-carb diet, the high-protein diet, the fat-flushing diet, the blood-type diet. . . . I could go on, but I like you too much.

Diet fads all work—for a while. You can achieve a certain weight doing all manner of silly things. But most are not sustainable over time, and some are downright

Voice of Success: "I Never Deprive Myself of Anything Now."

Michelle Friedson, midtwenties, removed 100 pounds over 1½ years

"I'd always been overweight. Since age 11, I was always on a diet. I've tried them all. I always felt deprived. I would do well, then a holiday or vacation would roll around, and I would start bingeing on whatever I'd been doing without. For instance, I was on a no-carb diet. Then I went on a cruise and gained 10 pounds in 10 days bingeing on carbs. When I returned home, I kept bingeing. The change came when I learned to see healthy eating as a way of life. I never deprive myself of anything now. Initially, I stopped the things I used to binge on like salty carbs and didn't go out to dinner until I could get my Mind, Mouth, and Muscle figured out. With Dr. Peeke's help, I discovered why I had been eating the way I was and learned to enjoy eating healthily and exercising. I found great health food at Trader Joe's and learned to find healthy options even when I eat out. Recently, I went on a cruise and didn't gain a pound!"

dangerous. The price you're paying in Body Dollars will bankrupt your mind and body. The mistaken assumption of diets is that you get weight loss fast by cutting corners. Usually, you feel like a lab rat. Also, severe calorie deprivation can cause a rebound in which you gain the weight back when you begin to eat "normally." Remember, your body does not want you to starve to death. When you restrict calories too much, it responds by slowing your metabolism to conserve its fat reserves. It becomes more efficient in absorbing nutrients (read: calories) so ultimately, you gain even more weight. Most important, you *decrease* the quality of your body—you lose muscle—when you're racing about on diet fads.

Fad diets also create a sense of deprivation, which leads to "cheating." The allure for the forbidden is very strong. In one study, scientists in Great Britain told 12 out of a group of 25 women to stay away from sugary snacks. Then they put all 25 in a room together with a load of sweets. Which group ate more? Yup, you guessed it.

The concept of quick-fix dieting implies that you're onto something that is short term and so, at some point, you will go back to "eating normally" again. What's up with that? If normal got you into this mess in the first place, why would you want to go back there?

Ultimately, fad diets are ineffective because they focus on weight as a number on a scale. That does not nor ever will work! Please hear this: No matter what fad diet you use, your weight loss is temporary. Two-thirds of the weight is regained within 1 year, and almost all is regained within 5 years. That's why, for the majority of people "trying to lose weight," yo-yo dieting or weight cycling is "normal"—rapid weight losses and equally rapid weight regains. That's bad. There's a link between weight cycling and high blood pressure, high cholesterol, and gall bladder disease. It's also not good mentally—weight cyclers tend to report depression and feelings of failure.

Until recently, the science of weight removal simply was not up to par. We didn't know what helped people really Cut the Fat and keep it off. So we were at the mercy of so-called "experts" hawking the latest fad. Folks, they are preying upon your emotions. Once you get the wake-up call that you are out of shape and overweight, you feel desperate. You want an end to your pain *right now*. Thus the demand for a quick fix. As a result, we've been spending tremendous Body Dollars (as well as heaps of actual dollars) in losing and gaining those same pounds. Actually, it's worse—because the rebound effect from dieting results in gaining *more* weight. This has got to stop.

⇒Fit to Live⇐
Cut the Fat and Trim the Tummy

"For many people, food feels nothing at all like a source of pleasure;
it feels like a minefield."
—MARION NESTLE

Those who are Fit to Live don't do fad diets. They choose a healthy eating plan and integrate it into a balanced lifestyle. To be Fit to Live, you need to concentrate not on the quantity of your body, but the quality. That means stop focusing only on weight. Instead, look at your *body composition*. Knowing how much fat you have and where it's located is key to not only becoming fit, but also to saving your own life. Remember that old Toxic Belly Fat problem?

Your body composition is made up of fat, muscle, and bone. You have control over the quantity and quality of all three factors. How much and what you eat, along with your physical activity and genetic pool, will determine what your body looks like.

You need to know your body composition, because excess body fat and not enough lean muscle not only makes us susceptible to all the diseases you've learned about, but also leads to a body that is overburdening the weight-bearing joints—the ankles, the hips, and the knees. You also need to know, because you can be a normal body weight with too much body fat *because* you don't have enough muscle mass. That means you don't have the metabolic power to burn calories efficiently, condemning yourself to a life of struggles with

Fascinating FAToid
Don't Pass On the Problem

More than half of teenaged girls and almost half of 9 to 11 year olds are on diets—or believe they should be. They're trying to take off the 40 pounds girls are supposed to put on between the ages of 8 and 14. Eighty-four percent of girls in a national survey believe they have to be thin to be popular. **Bottom line:** Let's be good role models and help our kids learn to become Nutritionally Fit to Live, for life.

excess body fat. The scale has deceived you into thinking you're in great shape because it's under a certain number. But you're still not Fit to Live to survive—*you just don't know it.* So lose the weight obsession and focus on body composition.

So what are some good body-fat numbers? Throughout a man's adult life, his body fat should be anywhere from 15 to 25 percent. As a man gets older, he may pick up a little bit more. But no man out there should be walking around with a body fat of 30 percent or greater. One big reason is that so much of that will be in the Toxic Belly Fat area.

It's different for women. As soon as we become adolescents, our body fat begins to shoot up from 12 to 15 percent to 18 to 25 percent. That body fat helps prepare a woman's body for pregnancy. Breasts, hips, buttocks, and thighs are all involved in providing the nutrients to feed a hungry baby.

A healthy 25- to 40-year-old woman should be anywhere from 20 to 25 percent body fat. (See "Ideal Body-Fat Ranges over the Life Span" below.) Pregnancy complicates the situation. Clearly, you try to aim for a 25-pound weight gain and get back to your prepregnancy weight. With each pregnancy, it's easy to pick up more body fat. That's why staying fit is so important. During her forties and into her fifties, a woman's body fat can increase somewhat. Up to the time of menopause, it's important to try to keep body fat as close to 25 percent as possible. After menopause, and through the sixties, seventies, and beyond, body fat may increase because muscle mass may fall. Therefore, the outside norm for body fat for older women is approximately 30 percent. However, it's really good for a woman to strive to keep as close to 25 percent as possible throughout her lifetime and under 30 percent if she can.

Unfortunately, most women have no idea that it is body fat they should be concentrating on. So, unbeknownst to them, while they've been struggling to keep their weight down through chronic restrictive dieting, their body fat has been creeping up. This lack of awareness frequently leads a woman to end up with a body-fat percentage equal to her age! I keep seeing 45-year-old patients with 45 percent body fat. When I tell them the number, they almost fall off the chair.

IDEAL BODY-FAT RANGES OVER THE LIFE SPAN

AGE	25–40 YR	40–55 YR	55+ YR
Men	15%–25%	15%–25%	<30%
Women	20%–25%	20%–27%	25%–30%

So consider this my heads-up to you. Pay attention to how much body fat you're carrying. (See "Track Your Journey" on page 133.) Women, if you're wearing too much body fat, you're increasing your risk for breast cancer. And the location of your body fat will determine how long you live—that Toxic Belly Fat thing.

> "No diet will remove all the fat from your body because the brain is entirely fat. Without a brain, you might look good, but all you could do is run for public office."
> —*Covert Bailey*

As men and women age, it's much easier to pick up fat around your belly area, especially the outside in a pooch extending from your belly button to your pubic area. This is a very normal redistribution of outer fat, which is caused primarily by the shift in sex hormones in both genders. There's no way to get around this, ladies and gentlemen. That little menopot (women) or manopot (men) is coming your way. You cannot eliminate it. Your job is to *minimize* it with your Fit to Live lifestyle.

As you learned in Chapter 1, you want to make sure the inner fat remains under control. Remember, women need to keep their waistline (tape measure across the belly button) less than 35 inches and men less than 40 inches. If you're over the limit, you're picking up Toxic Belly Fat deep inside the tummy, ramping up your risk for heart disease and diabetes.

That's why, when I talk about removing weight, I'm really talking about removing fat, particularly Toxic Belly Fat, and building muscle. I never talk about *losing* weight. *Losing* your keys is a bummer. You want to find them again. You don't want to *lose* fat and then plan on finding it again. You want to *remove* fat permanently. So from now on, use that word. It's a one-way ticket, signaling that these are lifelong, sustainable changes.

HIS AND HER WEIGHT REMOVAL

When you think about weight removal, you must take gender into account. The reality is that men drop weight faster than women do. Part of that is physiology, as you will learn shortly. But part has to do with the way they approach Cutting the Belly Fat. When I wrote *Body*-for-*LIFE for Women,* I turned my attention to the critical mental and physical differences between the genders that determined how they approached their weight management. That's when I realized that motivation looks very different for men and women.

What prompts men to drop weight is often a quantifiably specific health-related issue. And it's rarely accompanied by a lot of emotion. Governor Mike Huckabee exemplifies

> *"Dost thou think, because thou art virtuous, there shall be no more cakes and ale?"*
> —*William Shakespeare*

this. When asked what got him going on weight loss, he replied, "I didn't set out to lose weight. I wanted to be healthy. I wanted to be able to sprint across the governor's mansion without calling 911. I wanted to not have to take medicine for my diabetes."

Women are often driven by how they feel. They come in and say, "I feel terrible about myself. I saw myself in the class reunion picture, and I'm huge! . . . And oh, by the way, I have high blood pressure." I keep a box of tissues by the patient chair in my office. I've yet to have a man shed one tear; women are often grabbing tissue within the first 10 minutes.

Men are rooted in reality—they understand that it's really a numbers game: calories in, calories out. They just hop to it, create a goal, and get the job done. Like building a wood cabinet. Get the data you need, the equipment to do it, and hammer away.

Women too often ruminate and let their inner perfectionist rear its ugly head, along with the relentless self-critic (how could you let yourself get this fat?) and the procrastinator (tomorrow, next Monday). Women have a Mental Cuisinart; men have a Mental Machete. We need to start thinking more like the guys, ladies. Set a goal and just do it.

Male or female, how much body fat you can remove in what time frame depends on a number of factors:

1. Age. The younger you are, the easier it is. It's more challenging after the age of 40. The reasons involve everything from declining sex hormones to greater calorie-burning inefficiencies at the cellular level.

2. Gender. In addition to better attitudes, men take weight off faster because their greater muscle mass and less body fat makes it easier to burn calories faster. Also, male hormones allow men to grow existing muscle and build new muscle faster.

3. Genetics. Some people look at food and wear it, while others look at that same food and it combusts. The obesity gene will definitely make it more challenging to achieve your best weight and body composition, but you can do it. Remember that genetics loads the gun, but environment pulls the trigger. Use everything you learn here to make the best of it.

4. Everything else going on with your body. Are you taking medications like anti-inflammatory steroids or antidepressants, which cause weight gain? Do you have problem knees? These factors will influence how quickly you can shed weight.

5. Your body type. There are three: ectomorph (the string bean), endomorph (the fluffy potato), and mesomorph (the lean steak). Most people are a mix, and everyone has some good muscular and athletic tendency. So maximize your inner mesomorph and minimize your endomorph.

6. Ethnic differences. Asians have a disproportionate amount of Toxic Belly Fat relative to their normal weights. Hispanics often have Toxic Belly Fat as well as excess overall body fat. African Americans in general tend to have more muscle, and African American women tend to have a greater body-fat distribution in their lower body.

What are realistic goals for body-fat removal then? An obese woman (at least 50 pounds over healthy weight) who follows the Fit to Live plan should be able to remove 25 to 30 pounds of body fat in 12 weeks. An obese man can remove 30 to 40 pounds in the same period of time. If you have 20 to 25 pounds of fat to remove, 12 weeks should do the trick quite nicely.

The only caveat is that during those 12 weeks, life may throw a wrench into your well-planned program. You get a new deadline on a critical work project, your kid gets arrested, your partner becomes depressed, you break a leg. These things happen. What do you do?

It's hard, but you have to strive not to spend huge Body Dollars slipping into health-destructive habits under stress. Count on your old buddy A² and work around the challenge. For example, you can always lift upper-body weights while your leg is healing.

Above all, remember that permanent weight removal happens methodically. It's phased in piece by piece. There are two processes. One is *removing* excess body fat by burning more calories than you consume through eating less and moving more. The other one is *maintaining* the body composition you end up with. It takes time to create the body composition changes you're striving for. Once you do, it becomes 50 times easier to *sustain* because it's a part of you. The Body Dollars spent go down while your reserves go up.

Fascinating FAToid
Toxic Fat Gone for Good
Those who maintain weight removal for 2 to 5 years halve their risk of ever regaining. **Bottom line:** Embrace this as a non-negotiable lifestyle choice, and weight cycling disappears.

I've been studying the secrets of thousands of successful weight removers for many years, both my own patients as well as those who have been being tracked by the National Weight Control Registry. This is a group of over 6,000 people who have removed an average of 67 pounds and kept it off anywhere from 5 to 10 years. If you think you can't remove Toxic Belly Fat because you've been heavy your whole life, consider this: Half of the people in the registry were overweight as kids, and three-quarters had at least one overweight parent.

Based upon this unique study, and my years of working with overweight and obese men, women, and children, I've boiled down the key weight-removal success factors into five principles. When combined with the other elements of the Fit to Live plan, this template will give you a holistic, integrated approach to weight removal.

THE FIVE FIT TO LIVE PERMANENT WEIGHT-REMOVAL PRINCIPLES

1. Hunger and Appetite Must Work in Harmony

Many obese and overweight folks are terrified of hunger. One of my obese patients who had gastric bypass surgery—top weight 410, now 275—said that until the surgery, she had never felt hunger. Now, she's working through phases—panic, anxiety—learning not only that it is okay when hunger hits, but that it's a beautiful sign of a bodily need.

Food is body fuel. It's not for making you feel better when you've had a lousy day, a reward for working hard, or to be used as your own 24-hour, on-call therapist. If you are eating appropriate amounts of the right foods every 3 to 4 hours, chances are when the food demons call your name, it's about appetite (I want) rather than hunger (I need).

Hunger is a visceral, physical, primal, hardwired feeling. It could be manifesting itself as anything from a headache or sweats to those really embarrassing stomach noises or the shakes. Appetite drives you to an attractive food choice that is tasty and palatable and something that feels good in your mouth. Hunger answers the question, what do I need? I need breakfast. Appetite answers the question, what do I want? I want oatmeal and fruit and coffee. They're in harmony. That's the goal.

> "I've been on a diet for 2 weeks, and all I've lost is 2 weeks."
> —*Totie Fields*

When appetite goes off on its own, remind yourself "I can't possibly be hungry. I just ate an hour ago." Then quickly assess what's happening. Did someone just upset you? What are the emotions flowing through you? Anxiety, frustration, disappointment? How about that Toxic Stress trio—hopelessness, helplessness, and defeat? Take a deep breath, and realize that your need to inhale a mountain of chocolate or mashed potatoes is based not upon hunger but emotionally driven appetite.

2. Deprivation Is Out, Healthy Pleasures Are In

Deprivation is dangerous because it always leads to bingeing disasters. Never, ever, ever walk around feeling deprived. Instead—this is an order—incorporate healthy pleasures!

Voice of Success: "My Genetics Were Not My Destiny."

Hillary Buckholtz, 27, removed 120 pounds and has kept it off for 10 years

"From the time I was born, my mom was fixated on saving me from the pain she endured growing up. Mom was determined not to subject me to what her mother did to her with food and her weight—the preoccupation, surveillance, hiding, judging, shaming—THE GUILT. Yet despite her best efforts, she did the same thing as her mom and then some. The afternoons of my childhood are a montage of doctor visits. Therapists, psychiatrists, nutritionists, basement offices, university hospitals, treatment centers, scales, charts, calipers, folders, equations, fake plastic food models. At 5 feet 11 inches and 13 years old, my top weight was nearly 300 pounds.

"The summer before high school, I stepped into Dr. Peeke's office. What she laid out for me was too simple to argue with—I had a predisposition toward obesity, but my genetics were not my destiny. I could turn this thing around. And I did. Through humor and friendship and honesty, she taught me how to eat and move and handle stress. The weight loss is actually where the story begins. There is NOTHING PAST TENSE about losing weight!! This is something that takes daily work and focus—there is no graduation ceremony. Losing the weight was the easy part. Maintaining my weight loss and living through stresses and adapting to challenges of life—that's where things got really interesting. Now, I approach myself from a place of love and gentleness, rather than from a place of fear and punishment. I am actually a friend to myself, and I experience daily miracles and new freedoms beyond my wildest dreams."

Fascinating FAToid

The Danger Zone

The hour that most people blow it with eating is 4:30 p.m. **Bottom line:** Eat a balanced feeding every 3 to 4 hours, and you'll blow right past the midafternoon without health-destruction.

But incorporate them occasionally as treats and not every day. For instance, I might have a glass of wine during a Friday night dinner with friends, but I don't do it every night.

You can eat any food or drink as a healthy pleasure so long as it's a nonbingeable. We've talked about how to avoid bingeables, troublesome can't-have-just-one foods. Science has shown that the pleasure centers in some people's brains are particularly sensitive to appetizing foods, making them more vulnerable to bingeing. Remember what you learned in Chapter 5 about addictions. Tell your True Truth and completely avoid your bingeables.

3. If You Fail to Plan, You Plan to Fail

Folks who are successful at removing excess body fat and keeping it off all share one trait—they're good at planning. Because of this, thinking ahead to plan healthy meals and pack healthy snacks for work comes easily. They are not obsessively sitting around counting every calorie. Instead, they have a general idea about what works for them, based upon trial and error and refining over weeks and months of daily living. One study found that participants shed an average of 14 pounds simply by thinking about what they ate at lunch before eating an afternoon snack.

Planning actually takes three kinds of thinking: organization, step-by-stepness, and timeliness. You can learn each through daily activities. Strengthen organization by planning out a week of meals in advance and shopping for them on the weekend. Develop step-by-stepness by tracking your quantity of food with a food journal. Cultivate timeliness by keeping your self-made appointment to go to the grocery store or gym. Planning needn't be complicated. As you learned in the last chapter, successful losers eat a few *simple* high-quality meals.

Consistency is crucial here. Those who do best stick with it consistently, day in and day out, remembering the 80/20 rule: Do it right 80 percent of the time, leaving 20 percent for just being human. This is *not a diet* but a lifestyle that you humbly accept as necessary to become Fit to Live.

4. Become a Calorie Cheapskate

Successful losers are very physically active. They do, on average, an hour of activity a day, or about 2,800 calories of exercise a week. You'll be learning more about that in the next chapter. For now, remember when I talked about giving food value in Chapter 6? One way successful losers make food valuable is to think of it in terms of calories that must be spent in exercise. That can of soda—15 minutes on the treadmill. That piece of cake—45 to 60 minutes on the elliptical.

BYPASSING THE BODY

In 2004, there were 20,000 bariatric surgeries performed in the United States. In 2006, there were 200,000. That's an increase of 900 percent. I recommend bariatrics if you truly have significant, life-threatening medical conditions such as dangerous heart problems, high cholesterol, which is associated with being at least 100 pounds above your ideal body weight. And only after very close medical scrutiny, as well as a guarantee that before and after surgery, you'll have psychological counseling, nutritional guidance, and supervised physical activity.

This is drastic surgery, folks. The mortality rate for gastric bypass, the most common surgery, is 1 in 200. Four out of every 10 people have complications, and for 1 in 20, they're serious, including heart attacks, kidney failure, and strokes. Protein, vitamin, and mineral deficiency are common, which results in fatigue, weakness, and/or hair loss. Some people develop serious vision problems due to vitamin A deficiency in spite of taking supplements. One-third of patients develop gallstones. Vomiting affects up to 30 percent of patients.

As *Passing for Thin* author Frances Kuffel, who removed over 170 pounds naturally, put it, "Gastric bypass is GI surgery, not brain surgery. Once the surgery is done, you still have the same screwed-up notions about eating, self-esteem, and exercise as you walked in with." That's why, after about 18 months, some people are back to overeating. Bariatric surgery is no magic pill. It may be lifesaving for some people. Just remember, you still have to do exercise and watch the quality, quantity, and frequency of eating.

5. It's a Hero's Journey

In my experience, every person who removes weight permanently has an experience that's very much like the hero's journey in *Star Wars* or *Harry Potter*: They experience the stages of change as described in Chapter 2 and accept that this is a lifetime lifestyle approach. They found a guide for the journey (coach, mentor, teacher, or group), separated from their old environment, and were reborn into the Fit to Live way of living. Women tend to do it in groups; men by themselves with one guide. They all found quiet time to reflect on themselves and their habits—meditation, yoga, journaling, etc. And after they achieved their weight goal, success spurred them on to achieve other goals in their lives. That's where the Enjoy and Challenge levels come in. The more you understand that you are on a heroic journey, the more you can embrace it as the exciting and life-altering experience it is.

⇒Fit to Live Essentials⇐

Using your score from the "Are You Nutritionally Fit to Live?" test, you'll continue to build your individual program with the tips below. As in previous chapters, you'll begin according to your current level.

TO SURVIVE:

If you received a score of 0 to 6 on the test, focus your energy here first. Once you've mastered these, feel free to move up to the tips in "To Enjoy."

1. Eat Breakfast

This goes against your "dieting" behavior, right? You wake up, swear to diet, and the first thing you do is skip breakfast. But one of the things successful weight removers have in

Fascinating FAToid
Don't Go It Alone

Obese people who had counseling lost twice as much as those who did not. Phoning worked as well as face to face. **Bottom line:** However you get it, you do better when you get help. Be sure to check out www.drpeeke.com in the Mouth section for individual and group help.

common is that they eat a healthy breakfast. Having breakfast begins the natural rhythm of eating every 3 to 4 hours. Perhaps you've already exercised, and now your hunger and appetite are working harmoniously to guide

> "The first thing you lose on a diet is brain mass."
> —*Margaret Cho*

you to your oatmeal or kashi or omelet. Remember, feeling hungry for breakfast is a test. If you ate too much the night before, you won't be hungry in the morning. If you are, you did just fine.

2. Eat More for Lunch Than Dinner

I call this the "Aunt Eva factor" after my husband Mark's 92-year-old aunt. She's fit and spry and has a better memory than you and me, so listen up! Her biggest meal is lunch and then she eats very lightly for dinner. If you follow Aunt Eva's example, you will have *guaranteed* weight removal. Make lunch your main meal and then for dinner have voluminous vegetables and a serving of lean protein. It works like a charm.

3. Use Lean Protein to Cut Carb Cravings

Eating protein has been proven to curb hunger pangs and depress appetite, which results in eating fewer calories. So when you're hungry, turn to lean protein—low-fat mozzarella string cheese, hard-cooked egg whites, fat-free yogurt—to satisfy those pangs. You'll be less likely to find yourself inhaling an unthawed frozen cheesecake or gobbling a mountain of pasta.

4. Track Your Journey

People who are the most successful at permanently removing excess weight track their journey. There are a number of creative ways to do this. I recommend a weekly weighing and a monthly body-fat check. Buy one of those bathroom-looking scales that are body-fat analyzers. Some of them are quite fancy and actually give you a full breakdown of your muscle, bone, and fat. The basic ones cost no more than a very good scale ($60 to $110). I also recommend measuring your girth across your belly button, as well as your menopot (women) or manopot (men). You can add other parts of your body, but the belly girth is where it's at—less than 35 inches for women, less than 40 inches for men. Use the Body Composition Tracker in Appendix 2 to record your

Fascinating FAToid

Spice It Up

Spicy food may help you burn more calories because it generates body heat and therefore reduces the energy stored from eating. People who drank tomato juice with a dash of red pepper, for instance, reduced by 5 to 10 percent the amount of energy consumed from meals. **Bottom line:** This isn't a license to pig out, just to spice it up a bit. If nothing else, adding spice makes basic food more interesting!

measurements, or just write them in a simple notebook or on your computer. I don't care where it goes. Just keep track.

When you're beginning your Nutrition Fitness journey, you need to get a general idea about how much you're eating. As I described in Chapter 6, you can calculate your total calorie needs in a rough approximation. Then just pay attention. Read labels. Stick with recommended serving sizes. People who spend a little time tracking—even just in their head—approximate calorie intake remove more weight than folks who wing it. Steady food diarists even remove weight over the holidays, while others gain as much 500 percent more per week.

5. Use Your Clothes-o-Meter

If you're already where you should be in terms of size, pick a pretty tight and fitted piece of clothing to be your Clothes-o-Meter. Put it on once a week. If it's too tight, pay close attention to your eating and exercise for a bit. If it feels great, you're in balance.

For you folks who need to shed excess body fat, grab a piece of clothing that fits you snugly in your current size. If you're a 16, select the tightest 16 you have. Guys, if you're a belt size 44, then put it on and note the notch you're starting with. Any piece of clothing will work so long as it's fitted.

One of the best stories from my practice was when I met with an obese woman for the first time and asked her current size. Her answer was, "Elastic." Let's just say it'd been a while since she'd seen numbers. Whatever your size, I highly caution against wearing elastic. Elastic is trouble—you can put on 20 pounds and barely notice.

The Clothes-o-Meter is a terrific mind-body tool. You're not ignoring your physical self and staring at a piece of metal—the scale. Instead, you're feeling your body as you slip your jeans or belt on. It's a reality check. Down with dissociation and up with connecting mind and body!

TO ENJOY:

If you scored a 7 to 13 on the test, just take a quick look at the "To Survive" suggestions. If you feel you have them covered, you can start here.

1. Spread the Comfort

There's nothing wrong with comfort foods, but why should food hog all the comfort? I remember the day I bought my very first cashmere scarf. I felt rotten that day and needed something soft around me. Identify what you need and get it: comfort CDs, comfort socks, comfort flowers, comfort hug, comfort movie. This is about tuning in to what you need, rather than using food as the one-stop shop for comfort, reward, distraction, boredom, friendship, and stress reduction. When you meet your need directly, you'll enjoy your life more.

2. Relish the Next Size Down

I'm giving you a Peeke prescription to do some retail therapy. Don't wait until you hit your target. As soon as you are in the next smaller size, celebrate by getting rid of all your bigger sizes, and buy one thing in that new size. When you reach your healthiest body composition, give away all your big clothes, and visit your neighborhood tailor and get some favorite clothes taken in. Then, go out and slowly buy a new wardrobe. Make an appointment with a personal shopper (great for men as well as women). Don't keep opting for your overweight colors—navy blue, black, brown. These are "hide-it colors." Experiment with new colors and rejoice now that you have a fitter, leaner, and stronger body.

3. Celebrate Doing Things You Couldn't Do Before

I'm not talking about bungee jumping here. I'm talking about what seem to be small things but are in reality incredible accomplishments. Couldn't wrap a towel around you? Couldn't easily slip into the molded chairs at the movies? Couldn't get in and out of your car without grimacing with pain and discomfort? Celebrate and relish the signs that you are Cutting the Toxic Fat. Say goodbye to seat belt extenders. To elastic-waist pants. To those T-shirts that are so big, they could carry you to another state in a strong wind.

Fascinating FAToid
The Power of a Food Diary

People who write down everything they eat discover they underestimate how much they're eating by about 1,050 calories daily—that's an extra pound every 3½ days. **Bottom line:** Don't obsess, but do try to be aware of the number of calories you're consuming.

TO CHALLENGE:

If you scored a 14 to 20 on the test, just take a quick look at the "To Survive" and "To Enjoy" tips. If you feel you have them covered, you can start here.

1. Live Your Dreams

Your body composition is optimal, and you'll keep refining and monitoring it. Now, make a list of all the things you have wanted to do but were afraid to because you were hauling too much body fat around. Roller coasters at the park, walking or biking vacations in Europe, salsa dance lessons, martial arts, scuba diving, or mountain climbing. Get out there and sign right up. The win/win is that not only are you able to put that new body composition to the test, but also the goal helps you stay on track and reminds you to thoroughly enjoy the challenge.

2. Keep Chiseling Away at the Fat

Congratulations on shedding enough excess body fat to reach your belly size goal. How about putting some distance between you and the basic survival requirement for girth and body fat? Can you give me another ½ inch on your waistline? If you're just meeting your body-fat percentage requirement, cut your body fat down 1 or 2 percent more. This refining process puts more Body Dollars in reserve for that time in your life when you will need it.

3. Spread Your Body Dollar Wealth

At the challenge level, you've been accumulating lots of Body Dollar reserves. Like a successful financial advisor who's banked a fortune, how about sharing your knowledge? If friends, family members, or colleagues ask for help on their wellness journeys, give 'em a helping hand. Volunteer at the Y or a school and help teach kids about nutrition. Some Fit to Live folks have gone on to become real health and fitness teachers. It's amazing what can happen when you become fearless.

PART 3

Muscle: Are You Physically Fit to Live?

"Too many people confine their exercise to jumping to conclusions, running up bills, stretching the truth, bending over backward, lying down on the job, sidestepping responsibility, and pushing their luck."
—ANONYMOUS

This section addresses the question, Am I Physically Fit to Live? To Survive, to Enjoy, to Challenge—and to save my life? Stand up. Can you see your toes? Bend over and try to touch them. Should you care if you can do these things? You bet your life. First, if you can't see your toes, the only thing in the way is your belly. Your Girth Control dilemma is not just a technical issue but a life-threatening problem. You know by now that too much fat deep inside your belly ramps up your risk for heart disease, diabetes, and cancer. Second, if you can't get close to touching your toes without popping your hamstrings, then you're in trouble when you need to break a fall. You need flexibility, balance, and strength to prevent breaking bones, spraining ligaments, or banging your head on concrete.

In the Introduction, I said that if you'll let me, I'd help you save your life. To do that, you must become Physically Fit to Live in two ways. One is to minimize your Toxic Belly Fat to live your best life and decrease your chance of disease and disability. The other is to get strong enough to survive your daily life—to be able to catch yourself if you start to fall, crawl up stairs in an emergency, pick up and run with a pet or a child. With my Fit to Live Essentials, both objectives are achieved at the same time. You'll not only create the Body Dollar reserves in endurance, strength, flexibility, and balance to prevent or minimize life-threatening disasters, while trimming that belly, but you'll also have a body that is strong and flexible enough to enjoy your life. And that stronger body can help you challenge yourself to achieve dreams that will bring you an incredible sense of accomplishment and joy.

To begin, find out your current level of physical fitness. This assessment is meant to be done within your own living environment. No gym required! If you don't have stairs, find some in your neighborhood. Go outside to do the walking test. Choose the answer that best describes your capacity to do the activity: "Swimming in sweat" would be really hard or impossible; "Breaking a sweat" would be somewhat hard; and "No sweat!" would be really easy. If you can't do it at all, write a 0 as your score for that section.

ENDURANCE

You are in the basement when suddenly there is an explosion and fire. To save your life, you must bolt up the stairs and get to safety. That requires cardio endurance. The following will test your Fit to Live endurance level:

1. Without holding onto the railings, can you climb 20 stair steps in 40 seconds?
   a. "Swimming in sweat"
   b. "Breaking a sweat"
   c. "No sweat!"

2. Time yourself in a 1-mile fast-paced walk on a flat surface. Compare your time against the "1-Mile Walk" chart in Appendix 1.
   a. Slower than you should be or can't do it at all
   b. At age and gender level
   c. Above average for age and gender

3. Time yourself in a 1.5-mile run on a flat surface. Compare your time against the appropriate "1.5-Mile Run" chart in Appendix 1.
   a. Slower than you should be or can't do it at all
   b. At age and gender level
   c. Above average for age and gender

Scoring:

1.   a, 0; b, 1; c, 2
2.   a, 0; b, 1; c, 2
3.   a, 0; b, 1; c, 2

Add up your score and check the key below.

0 to 1: Fit to Survive. Under normal circumstances, you manage all right. But being Fit to Live means being able to move quickly up stairs and past other obstacles when you face an emergency. Unless you make a commitment to getting in better shape, you're putting yourself in jeopardy. Read on to discover a game plan for success.

2 to 4: Fit to Enjoy. You're starting from a solid place—in this situation you should be able to make it to safety without much problem. Now the challenge is to get yourself into good enough shape to help anyone else who might be down there, like a child or elderly parent. Find out how in this chapter.

5 to 6: Fit to Challenge. You'll be able to bring yourself—and whoever needs your help—to safety in no time flat. Read on to find out how to strengthen your endurance even more.

STRENGTH

You and your child or grandchild are out alone in a deserted park. She's racing around and bumps into you. You both go down. You're just banged up but she's twisted her ankle. You've got to get yourself up and then you have to carry her (she weighs 40 pounds) to safety and get help. That takes strong arms, legs, and core (abdomen and back). The following will test your Fit to Live strength level:

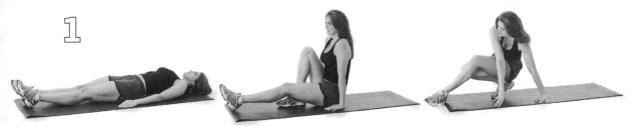

From a full standing position, get down flat on the floor. Can you get up again with no help?

a. "Swimming in sweat"
b. "Breaking a sweat"
c. "No sweat!"

2

Count how many times you can stand up from a chair with your arms folded across your chest in 30 seconds. Can do at least 8?

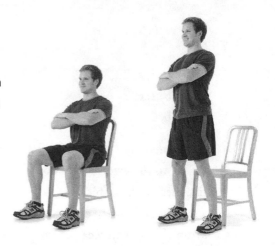

    a. "Swimming in sweat"
    b. "Breaking a sweat"
    c. "No sweat!"

3

Count how many pushups you can perform in 1 minute. Women, with bent legs; men, straight. Compare your results against the "Dynamic Strength Test" chart in Appendix 1.

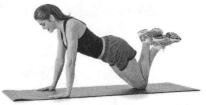

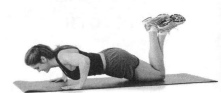

    a. Less than you should be able to do or not at all
    b. At age and gender level
    c. Above average for age and gender

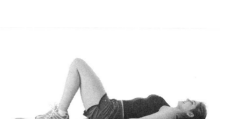

From a standing position (feet shoulder width apart, hands at the waist), squat down to a seated position.

Your back should remain upright, your knees should be over your toes on descend. Return to starting position. Repeat 10 times with good form.

    a. "Swimming in sweat"
    b. "Breaking a sweat"
    c. "No sweat!"

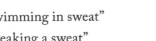

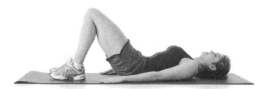

Lie flat on your back with knees bent. Imprint your lower back toward the floor (tilt the pelvis, bringing your hip bone toward your ribs). Repeat 10 times.

    a. "Swimming in sweat"
    b. "Breaking a sweat"
    c. "No sweat!"

6

Lie flat on your back with knees bent. Imprint the lower back toward the floor.

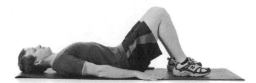

Lift your buttocks off the floor to form a "bridge." As you hold the bridge position, take one leg straight out, keeping your knees together. Hold for 5 seconds. Switch legs. Repeat the cycle 5 times.

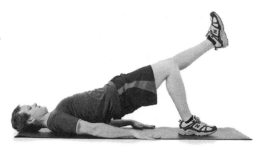

    a. "Swimming in sweat"
    b. "Breaking a sweat"
    c. "No sweat!"

7

Lie flat on your stomach with elbows bent by your side and your hands in a fist position.

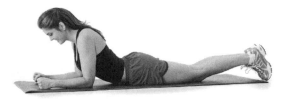

Take a deep breath and lift your stomach off the floor while keeping knees in contact with the floor. Hold the plank for 30 seconds. Return to the starting position.

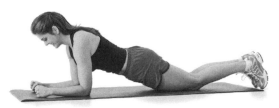

    a. "Swimming in sweat"
    b. "Breaking a sweat"
    c. "No sweat!"

Scoring:

1.	a, 0; b, 1; c, 2	5.	a, 0; b, 1; c, 2
2.	a, 0; b, 1; c, 2	6.	a, 0; b, 1; c, 2
3.	a, 0; b, 1; c, 2	7.	a, 0; b, 1; c, 2
4.	a, 0; b, 1; c, 2		

Add up your score and check the key below.

0 to 4: Fit to Survive. Your Body Dollar reserves are low. At your current fitness level, some situations requiring physical strength will be very difficult, if not impossible, for you. Read on to find out how you can build the strength you need to pick up a small child or pet. Not only will it make you and your loved ones more secure, you'll also feel great!

5 to 9: Fit to Enjoy. This challenge may leave you huffing and puffing, but the bottom line is you should be able to get your child or grandchild the help she needs. Read on to find out ways to build the strength you need to pick up heavy objects with ease.

10 to 14: Fit to Challenge. Great news! Not only will you be able to carry a small child or pet to safety, you'll also be able to help out an adult who needs a hand—say, your elderly mother or a friend who twists her ankle while skiing. Read on for more ways to build on your great foundation of strength.

FLEXIBILITY AND BALANCE

You're standing right by the tracks, waiting for the subway. Someone hurrying behind you rudely pushes you to go past. If you lose your balance, you will fall down onto the tracks and may be seriously hurt or killed. If you're flexible and strong and have good balance, you're more likely to stop the fall or minimize any damage. This test will gauge your Fit to Live flexibility and balance level:

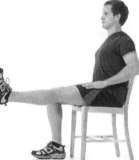

1

Sit on the edge of a chair with one leg extended out front and the other leg bent.

Reach forward toward your extended leg. Can you touch your toes? If not, can you come within 4 inches if you're a man? Or 2 inches if a woman?

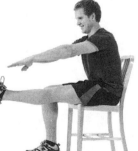

    a. "Swimming in sweat"
    b. "Breaking a sweat"
    c. "No sweat!"

2

Lie flat on your back.

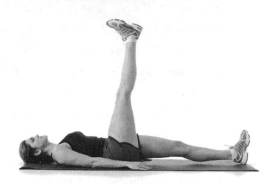

Raise one leg (knees straight) toward the ceiling.
Check how high you were able to raise your leg
without bending your opposite knee or arching your
lower back. Can you bring your leg to a 90-degree
angle?

a. "Swimming in sweat"
b. "Breaking a sweat"
c. "No sweat!"

3

With one hand reaching over the shoulder and one up the
middle of the back, have a friend measure the number of inches
between the extended middle fingers. If you're a man, can you
get them to touch or come within 4 inches? If you're a woman,
can you get them to touch or get within 2 inches?

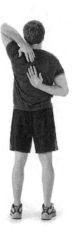

a. "Swimming in sweat"
b. "Breaking a sweat"
c. "No sweat!"

4

Sit against a wall with your legs crossed,
forearms flat against the wall.

Raise your arms toward the ceiling. Can you get
them all the way up without arching your back or
losing contact with the wall?

    a. "Swimming in sweat"
    b. "Breaking a sweat"
    c. "No sweat!"

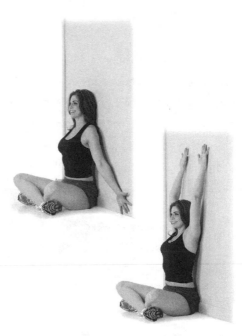

5

From a standing position, arms to the side, raise one foot.
Time how long you can hold the position without losing
your balance. Switch sides. Can you do 10 seconds on
both sides?

    a. "Swimming in sweat"
    b. "Breaking a sweat"
    c. "No sweat!"

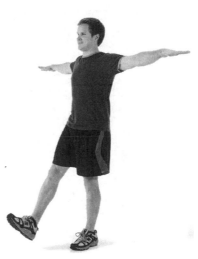

6

From a standing position, arms to the side, raise one foot and both arms overhead. Close your eyes. Time how long can you hold the position without losing your balance. Switch sides. Can you do 20 seconds or better on each side?

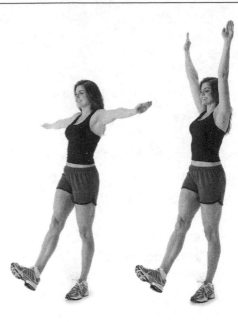

    a. "Swimming in sweat"
    b. "Breaking a sweat"
    c. "No sweat!"

7

From a standing position, lift one foot off the floor. Hop forward with the opposite leg. Repeat 5 times with each leg without touching the raised foot on the floor.

    a. "Swimming in sweat"
    b. "Breaking a sweat"
    c. "No sweat!"

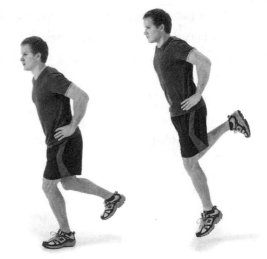

Scoring:
    1.   a, 0; b, 1; c, 2
    2.   a, 0; b, 1; c, 2
    3.   a, 0; b, 1; c, 2
    4.   a, 0; b, 1; c, 2
    5.   a, 0; b, 1; c, 2
    6.   a, 0; b, 1; c, 2
    7.   a, 0; b, 1; c, 2

Add up your score and check the key below.

0 to 4: Fit to Survive. You may not think that having tight, stiff muscles could put your life in jeopardy. But as this example shows, flexibility is just as important a survival skill as strength or endurance. Like many Americans, you have a lot of work to do in this department, so read on for exercises that will free your muscles and calm your mind.

5 to 9: Fit to Enjoy. You are probably flexible enough to avert disaster in this situation. However, a solid program of yoga and other forms of stretching will not only enhance your preparedness for an emergency but also bring a new level of ease and comfort to your body—and your life! Read on for more information.

10 to 14: Fit to Challenge. You have the flexibility and balance of a zen master—and this will serve you extremely well throughout your life. Your body responds quickly and agilely to life-threatening situations, and you enjoy a level of ease and comfort in everything you do—from walking or gardening to sitting at the computer—that most Americans cannot even fathom. Read on to find out how to further release tension and unlock tightness in tricky spots.

You've now assessed how Physically Fit to Live you are by evaluating your performance in the three key Muscle areas: Endurance, Strength, and Flexibility and Balance. Your individual scores tell you where you stand in that particular area and highlight the areas with the greatest potential for improvement. Your goal is to take any Survival level scores at work to achieve the Enjoy levels. If you're already at Enjoy, then take yourself on and try some of the Challenge exercises and see if you can achieve that level of physical fitness.

You may notice that you'll always have better endurance than strength, or vice versa. Just aim to improve your score in each category and then maintain yourself at the Enjoy level, and pushing your envelope when you want with the Challenge level. You'll use these scores to guide you through the entire Muscle plan in a balanced way as you continue to build a leaner and stronger body.

Bottom-Line Results from Becoming Physically Fit to Live to Enjoy

■ You'll save your life, and potentially other people's as well, if faced with a life-threatening accident or event requiring reserves of physical strength and stamina.

■ You'll reduce an overweight or obese waistline 2 to 3 inches per month until you reach less than 35 inches for women and less than 40 inches for men.

■ You'll cut up to 1 to 3 pounds of excess Body Fat (women) or up to 3 to 4 pounds of Body Fat (men) per week until you've reached your Body-Fat Percentage Goal and will keep it off.

■ You'll cut your risk of dying young by 25 percent and live, on average, 8 to 9 years longer.

■ If your blood sugar is high, you'll cut your risk of developing type 2 diabetes by more than 50 percent. If you have a family history and are disease-free so far, you can cut your risk of developing it by more than 40 percent.

■ You'll reduce your risk of heart attack by 65 to 90 percent and also reduce your risk of strokes; colon, prostate, pancreatic, and breast cancers; osteoporosis; and impotence.

■ You'll build 3 pounds of muscle in 12 weeks, increase your metabolism by 7 percent, improve your ability to use glucose fuel in your blood by 25 percent, and increase bone mass by 1 to 3 percent.

■ If you have arthritis, you'll reduce joint swelling and pain. If you don't, it can help prevent it from happening.

■ If you're a menopausal woman, you will relieve hot flashes and headaches by 50 percent.

■ You'll save $2,200 a year on medical bills if you're over 50.

■ If you're moderately depressed, you'll relieve your symptoms by 50 percent (which is equivalent to taking antidepressants) and get increased feelings of happiness, well-being, self-esteem, and confidence.

■ You'll sleep better while preventing and potentially reversing sleep apnea.

■ You'll reduce the risk of Alzheimer's by up to 60 percent and improve overall brain function, including memory and attention.

■ You'll likely delay by 12 years the onset of disabilities associated with aging.

CHAPTER 8

Sweatin' the Body

"A vigorous 5-mile walk will do more good for an unhappy but otherwise healthy adult than all the medicine and psychology in the world."
—PAUL DUDLEY WHITE

C ould you run down 10 or 20 flights of emergency stairs to save your life? Or race to catch a beloved child who's about to step into oncoming traffic? Are you sure? After having taken the endurance part of the Physically Fit to Live assessment, you might have had a rude awakening. That's okay. I'm going to teach you some basics so that when you need to walk or run to save your life, you'll have the reserves to pull it off. And remember, you're whittling away at your Toxic Belly Fat as well.

Endurance is created by cardiovascular fitness, also known as aerobic fitness. That's all about getting our blood pumping and hearts and lungs working. It's about doing any activity that requires you to suck up that oxygen and utilize it to get those muscles rocking and rolling. Unfortunately in America, too many of us don't have the reserves we need. Outside of a few professions, our bodies are only brain carriers—they carry around the gray matter that generates our income. In fact, our cardio fitness levels have been steadily declining

Fascinating FAToid

Cardio Can Control Colds

The risk of catching a cold dropped significantly in postmenopausal women who were doing daily cardio (walking, biking) and continued to drop more as time went on. **Bottom line:** Regular physical activity boosts immune function.

every decade since the '70s. Yikes! This is not good. Cardio fitness helps reduce Toxic Belly Fat and Toxic Belly Fat Syndrome factors such as high cholesterol, blood pressure, and insulin resistance. It also reduces bone loss in aging and creates the physical endurance we need for those out-of-the-blue emergencies. Not to mention the great mind effects like reducing stress and depression!

In this chapter, you'll learn easy and basic ways to get the old heart pumping on a regular basis. But first, we'll look at why you must humbly accept that, from now on, you've got to make the time to move.

⇨Our Toxic Lifestyle⇦
Exercise, What Exercise?

"A bear, however hard he tries, grows tubby without exercise."
—POOH'S LITTLE INSTRUCTION BOOK

Throughout most of human existence, our living environment made the local gym look like a walk in the park. We had to move to survive. Hunter/gatherers roamed and ran just to score food, and even when we became farmers, work was still very physical. If we wanted breakfast, there's the barn. Knock yourself out. Go milk a cow and then work it out with the chickens and eggs. You want to go to school? It's 3 miles that way.

For thousands of years, the work most human beings did was physically intense. Then we stopped moving. How many of us, aside from athletes and construction workers, do something physical for work? To make matters worse, as we saw earlier, along came TV and then video games and the Internet. And we began to spend lots of time with these toys, time we used to spend moving.

Researchers started making the physical fitness–health connection in the '60s. That's when my colleague Ken Cooper, MD, founder of the Cooper Aerobics Center, proved for the first time that regular aerobic activity prevented the development of a wide variety of diseases and that it is crucial to maintain adequate physical fitness levels throughout your life to maintain independence, reduce the chance of disability, and/or minimize disabilities' effects.

Our activity levels have been steadily declining for the past 30 years. For the majority of us, moving the body now means *driving,* and we do so much of that, we couldn't run if our lives depended on it. We now spend five times as many minutes driving as doing any non-work-related physical activity.

The Centers for Disease Control and Prevention guidelines for recommended cardio activity are moderate-intensity activities (brisk walking, biking, vacuuming) that cause small increases in breathing or heart rate for 30 minutes a day, 5 days a week, or vigorous activity (running, aerobics, or anything that causes large increases in breathing or heart rate) 20 minutes a day at least three times a week. On average, 60 percent of us aren't getting the recommended amounts, and about one-quarter of people do *no* physical activity at all. (In some Southern states, almost one-third of people get no exercise at all, and in Puerto Rico, that number is 45 percent!) Women are less active than men, and activity in general declines with age. In addition, nearly half of young people ages 12 to 21 aren't getting the required amounts, with physical activity dropping dramatically at adolescence.

And guess what, people? Those guidelines are really not enough. They don't include enough strength training or stretching or core or balance work (more on that in the next two chapters). They also don't account for the research from the National Weight Control Registry that found that successful losers did 60 minutes of exercise a day to both remove weight and keep it off. You can't remove weight by just eating right. In primate research,

Fascinating FAToid

Turn Off and Step Out

TV viewers are 47 percent less likely to walk 10,000 steps than nonwatchers. Scientists now know that for every hour of TV you watch, you reduce the number of your steps by 144. Since the average person now watches 8 hours a day, that's 1,152 fewer steps. **Bottom line:** Tune out and turn on to the joy of moving that magnificent body of yours.

Fascinating FAToid

Too Much Butt on Chair

The desktop computer started showing up on secretaries' desks in the early '80s. It got rid of the need, for all intents and purposes, to get up and go get files in a cabinet. The elimination of that one motion, day after day, was the equivalent of a 15-pound weight gain per year! **Bottom line:** We have to make movement intentional because we don't have to do it anymore.

it was found that sedentary monkeys got fat and active ones stayed thin, *regardless of how much food either group was eating.* Even the researchers were shocked, concluding that it's not so much how much we're eating but a lack of activity that makes folks fat.

Kids are as bad off as adults. High schoolers' enrollment in daily physical education classes was only 33 percent in 2005. Almost one-third of states do not require phys ed for students until high school. Nearly one-quarter of states allow students to receive gym credit for *online courses*. Yes, you read that right. This, at the same time that an international study concluded that children should have 90 minutes of daily physical activity.

Heart disease risk factors such as high cholesterol, high blood pressure, and insulin resistance start in early childhood, and physical activity at the 90-minute level reduces these factors, particularly insulin resistance. This may be particularly important to girls. Exercise when young can lower hormone levels and perhaps delay the onset of menstruation. That's good, because girls who don't get their periods until 13 or 14 have a lower risk of breast cancer throughout their lifetimes. Increased physical activity also lowers body fat in girls, which also helps reduce breast cancer risk.

Unfortunately, it's the people who could benefit the most who are moving the least. Exercise has been shown to cut type 2 diabetes risk by 50 percent. But among people at risk of developing it, those who were thinner; less depressed, stressed, or anxious; or more confident in their ability to exercise were more likely to do so. In other words, those who would benefit the most were *less* likely to do it. This is why it's so important to get the whole Fit to Live lifestyle going. When you're Cutting through your Mental Fat and getting Nutritionally Fit, you're more likely have the drive to do what you need to become Physically Fit to Live. And when you move, you'll be less depressed, stressed, and anxious, and more confident and happy. They're all exquisitely interrelated.

⇒Fit to Live⇐
Use It and You Won't Lose It

"I run because it's my passion and not just a sport. Every time I walk out the door, I know why I'm going where I'm going, and I'm already focused on that special place where I find my peace and solitude."
—SASHA AZEVEDO

Let's dispel an important myth. You're supposed to get fat and fall apart as you age. Wrong. As I explained in the opening of this book, the National Institute on Aging has clearly said that so many of what we thought were the symptoms of aging are actually the symptoms of *disuse*. Most 100-year-olds are very active people. They're not spending the whole day sitting around in a rocking chair staring at the wall. Instead, they walk, climb stairs, push, pull, and lift all day long. And this activity keeps 'em sharp and smart—and Alert and Vertical. Science has already shown that physical activity has a powerful effect on maintaining optimal brain function, including the prevention of dementias such as Alzheimer's. So let's get going!

THE FIVE FIT TO LIVE CARDIO PRINCIPLES

1. Cardio Creates Body Dollar Reserves

Imagine you're 30, not significantly overweight or obese, and you walk a mile. How much of your aerobic work capacity are you using? About 20 percent. That means it's real easy to

Fascinating FAToid
Not Moving Will Cost You

Lack of exercise is responsible for a quarter million deaths in the United States every year. In men, low aerobic fitness was a greater risk factor in dying than any other, including smoking and high blood pressure. In women, it was third, after diabetes and smoking. **Bottom line:** You can't afford not to move.

Fascinating FAToid
Avoiding Disability by Moving

Only 16 percent of normal or underweight people have arthritis, but more than 30 percent of obese Americans have it. And one-third of those say they have limitations in their activities as a result. **Bottom line:** Exercise has been proved to help prevent arthritis. The more you move, the more you'll take the weight off and reduce your pain and disability.

do—you're barely cracking a sweat. If in that moment, you had to run for your life, you'd have 80 percent reserves to rock and roll with.

Now you hit 50 and beyond, and guess what happens? Your aerobic work capacity begins to decrease and continues to decrease every decade *no matter what shape you're in.* It's just a function of aging. It happens to Olympians. It happens to slouch potatoes. If you're in great shape to start with, the decline still leaves you with plenty of Body Dollar reserves. If you're unfit, you just went from no reserves to Body Dollar debt.

Now imagine you're 70. Your aerobic work capacity is in the range of 50 to 80 percent, leaving you with only 30 to 50 percent in reserves for an emergency. You're really putting it out there to walk a mile let alone break into a sprint to save your life.

You think this is only a problem for older or overweight folks? It's hitting everyone right now. A woman in her forties broke down in my office the other day because she doesn't have the reserves to play tennis with her 14-year-old daughter. If this is true for you, what happens when your capacity declines as you age?

Here's the good news—no matter what shape you're in, no matter what your age, you can increase your cardio fitness and create a Body Dollar reserve. It doesn't matter if you are disabled, if you are suffering from a disease. Just start where you are. It's no different than putting money away for your kids' college tuition or for your retirement. The more

Fascinating FAToid
How about Sex as an Incentive?

Middle-aged men who became and stayed aerobically fit report a better sex life in terms of stamina and orgasms. **Bottom line:** Guys, if you were waiting for a reason, here's a hot one!

aerobically Fit to Live you become, the more Body Dollars you're banking to stay alive the longest you can with the greatest amount of high quality and joy in your life. *That's* what movement is really about!

2. Moving More Every Day Is Non-Negotiable

Okay, folks. We have to get over this resentment about the "one more thing" in an already jam-packed schedule. You have to move to save your life. You have to move to live long and well. You have to move to become fit to survive, enjoy, and challenge.

I wish there was a perfect environment within which to move. Perhaps a large comfy gym in everyone's home. Or maybe I could just put you all on farms and let you work it all off in sweat as you tried to survive on the plains. But, alas, it's the 21st century, and we have to come up with creative ways to do this. Use the outdoors and sports as much as possible. But when you can't, there are machines. Just get it done.

3. Movement Ends Mind-Body Dissociation

When you move, you stop dissociating from your body. One day, an overwhelmed mom came to see me. At 40, she rarely ever exercised and was feeling tired and depressed. She said, "Look at my body. I thought I was eating okay, but I don't feel good. I'm not over-weight, so I don't understand why I look and feel so bad." When I did her body composition, it showed that she'd been fooled by the scale. Her weight was normal, but her body fat was 33 percent, when 25 percent or less would be the norm. Why? Because she never used her body except to get in and out of her car.

I read her the riot act, saying, "You've got another 60 years to go. You've got to have the body that will cart your wonderful mind through the rest of it. Here's a pedometer. I want you to walk 10,000 steps a day."

She said, "Walking?" as if it were a foreign concept. "Where do I walk?"

"You have a neighborhood," I responded.

She started walking. A few weeks into her new program, I got a phone call. "I've gotta tell you the most amazing thing!" she said excitedly. "I was walking, and I felt sweat going down my thigh, right behind my knee. I love this walking!"

I replied, "Welcome to your body!"

> "The mind's first step to self-awareness must be through the body."
> —*George Sheehan*

Voice of Success: "You Can Expect More and Do More!"

Don Miller removed 40 pounds of Body Fat

"I had a coronary bypass in 2006 and got serious about becoming Fit to Live. I did the aerobics and weight training in Dr. Peeke's plan, dropped the weight, and got back to a fine level of fitness. Then I developed a non-life-threatening heart problem that left me breathless. The doctors say to slow down to deal with it. I'm not willing to do that. It's dangerous to live with low reserves. I might need reserves to deal with a family crisis, like the death of a loved one, or a business crisis, like having to go back and redo my company that I'm retired from. You need stamina for that. So I'm keeping the physical fitness up. I'm not going gently into that good night. As you get older, lots of physicians say, 'Well, what can you expect at your age?' You can expect more and do more!"

4. Medicate with Movement

If you have anxiety, depression, heart disease, cancer, diabetes, or an "-itis," which means "inflammation of," like arthritis, *medicate with movement!* Right now, because most of us are moving so little, we're not getting the natural painkillers and feel-good hormones our bodies produce when we get moving. Instead, we're medicating with drugs, alcohol, shopping, bad sex, and chocolate chip cookies. Which only compounds our problems in the long run. Because of the wonderful Mind-Muscle effects of movement, you'll not only feel better due to the release of mood and confidence elevators— serotonin, beta-endorphins, noradrenalin—but you'll be building those lifesaving Body Dollars.

Be inspired by my patient Betty Lawson, a breast cancer survivor. This 62-year-old had all her lymph nodes under her arms removed and must wear a special glove when at altitude. But that hasn't stopped her from climbing mountains, or, as I write this, walking in her eighth New York Marathon. She recently sent me an article about a guy with arthritis who's had 20 joint operations, including eight for replacement hips and knees, who's a mountain climber. She and he keep at it because moving makes them feel better. It can for you too.

5. Concentrate on What You Can Do, Not on What You Can't

I know that so many of you break out into hives at the thought of moving because you're immediately creating a litany of things you can't do. And the older you get, the longer the list is. Aching knees, bad backs, stiff necks, swollen joints can happen to anyone whether you've been an athlete or a couch potato. They're part of the cost of aging. Often these are then joined by the Toxic Stress of hopelessness, helplessness, and defeat. "I've always been a runner, and now my knees are shot." Come on and show us your best A²-ing. Start biking or swimming or rowing. Remember what Darwin said—it's those who can adapt that survive. "It hurts too much. I can only do half the exercises." Hey, half is a heck of a lot better than nothing! Concentrate on what you *can* do. The mathematical probability of aching somewhere on your body increases precipitously after the age of 45. So do what you can, given disabilities, stay consistent, and be proud of your achievement.

⇒Fit to Live Essentials⇐

Using your score from the first part of the "Are You Physically Fit to Live?" test, you'll continue to build your individual program with the tips below. As in previous chapters, you'll begin according to your current level.

TO SURVIVE:

If you received a score of 0 to 1 on the endurance test, focus your energy here first. Once you've mastered these, feel free to move up to the tips in "To Enjoy."

Fascinating FAToid

Movement Is Good Medicine

If you're obese or overweight, you'll improve your odds of surviving breast cancer if you develop it within a year of beginning exercising. Cardio conditioning can also help cancer patients deal with the side effects of chemo, particularly nausea, vomiting, and weight loss or gain. And doing aerobic exercise when you have colorectal cancer substantially reduces your risk of death from it or other causes. **Bottom line:** Work with your doctor to see how to incorporate increased physical activity to improve your healing and lower your risk for disease.

1. Cut the Excuse Fat and Take the Non-Negotiable Pledge

As you might guess, I've heard the whole laundry list of excuses: I don't have time; I'm too tired; it's boring; I don't feel like it; the kids are out of school for the summer; my mother broke her wrist; I'm on a deadline. I know it's hard. But do you want to live long and well? Have the life you deserve? Be fit to save your life? Well then, you're going to have to Cut the Excuse Fat and make daily movement non-negotiable.

Going to work is non-negotiable. Taking a shower is non-negotiable. Feeding your kids is non-negotiable. Your physical fitness needs to be also. From now on, moving is a non-negotiable item that you *humbly accept* as a part of life. Okay?

Of course, the more complicated your life is, the more creative you have to be. Kids make it more difficult. Do it first thing in the morning before the kids are up. Take the kids with you. Do it in the evening on a treadmill or stationary bike in front of the TV. Traveling? Bring along your sneakers and walk at the airport, up the stairs at the hotel, the park outside your window. If Condoleezza Rice, who flies 24,000 miles a month, can do it every day—and she does—so can you.

Do you keep your commitments to others? Of course. So now I want you to commit to yourself with the Cut the Excuse Fat, Non-Negotiable Pledge: I promise to move every day, rain or shine.

2. Burn 300 to 400 Calories a Day

Everyone says exercise for 30 minutes, 45 minutes, 90 minutes. Forget about time. Aim to burn 300 to 400 calories deliberately every day. If you're someone who needs to remove excess body fat, especially Toxic Belly Fat, then there's absolutely no question

Fascinating FAToid

No Time Is No Excuse

Fifty-seven percent of us say we exercise, but 70 percent know we need to do more, and 25 percent say we have "no time for physical activity." But the truth is, we have time, we're just choosing to do other things with it: We spend nine times as many minutes watching TV or movies as we do on all leisure-time physical activities combined. Nine times, people. **Bottom line:** You can make the time. You can even do it in front of the TV.

AVOID THESE AEROBIC NO-NOS

1. Leaning on that treadmill or elliptical. That's cheating. Plus, it's bad for your back. Stand up straight and hold on lightly.
2. Reading or talking on the cardio equipment. You're probably not getting your heart rate up enough.
3. Walking with weights. It can cause stress factures and give you an awkward stride. Do your strength training separately.
4. Trying to burn all your calories on the weekend. You'll be too sore on Monday. Plus you aren't getting the consistent conditioning that leads to maximum success. Aim for the 400 a day, especially if you want permanent fat reduction.
5. Pushing yourself too hard to start. You can hurt yourself and then give up. Remember, small steps yield big results.

it's got to be at least 400. Now, that's an average. One day it may be 200 calories, the next one 600.

What does it take to do that? Strap on a pedometer and get in 10,000 steps a day. Every mile you walk is about 100 calories, and 2,500 steps is roughly 1 mile, so 10,000 is approximately 4 miles and 400 calories. (It's actually a little more complicated than that, but it's a good rough estimate.)

You don't have to do all the steps at once. Divide up the miles during the day. Park a mile from your office and walk to and from. You're halfway there. The treadmill, stationary bike, rower, pool, or the elliptical at the gym are all wonderful cardio options, plus they have the advantage of tracking calories burned for you. They also keep you out of the cold and the rain and the snow.

To make it easier, try this. Remember how you named your Mental Fat in the Mind section: my mother-in-law pounds, my micromanaging boss pounds, my loneliness pounds? Close your eyes right now and imagine cans of fuel hanging off your body wherever you have excess fat. There you are, clanking along with all this excess fuel. Every time you do your cardio, imagine you're burning one of those cans. Toss it off, along with the Mental Stress that put it there. Bye-bye college pounds, divorce pounds, boredom pounds. Doesn't that feel better? Less clankin' goin' on!

3. Smell the Sweet Success from 6 Weeks

When they finally get the movement message, so many folks want to go out there and run like a Kenyan on day one. Then they give up when they either injure themselves or are in pain from exhaustion. Small steps lead to big results. That means you must be patient and persistent. If 10,000 steps is challenging for you, build up over 6 weeks.

Here's how: Using your pedometer, figure out how many steps you're walking on a typical day. Then add 500 to 1,000 steps a day per week. For instance, let's say you start out at 3,500. Adding another 500 every day or so, you'll be up to 6,500 at the end of the first week. Even if you average 5,000 steps that first week, you're a success because it's more than your starting point. Then add another 500 to 1,000 a day the second week. You'll have 4,000-step days, and you'll have 12,000-step days. Just stay in the game and be as consistent as you can. Once you get up to 10,000, do everything you possibly can to hold onto that level.

If you're an absolute beginner, you've probably been doing the 10,000 steps on flat ground. When you can do that easily, up the intensity by putting a little high step in your walking so that it's brisk. Then find a hill and/or increase your speed.

This 6-week buildup is applicable to any cardio you want to do. If you're a beginner, start out slower; burn 100 to 200 calories every day over the first week or so, and then increase each week until you reach your daily 400-calorie goal. Any walking you also do during the day is frosting on the cardio cake that just helps you Cut that Body Fat more efficiently.

4. Increase Your Activities of Daily Living

To burn those 400 calories, in addition to walking, find ways to increase your activities of daily living. Stairs at home and work are a good thing. Use 'em to Cut your Mental and Physical Fat. Walk around for a few minutes at least once an hour, and by the end of the day, you've accrued lots of Toxic Belly Fat–burning activity.

All this activity of daily living is lifesaving. By observing folks between 70 and 82 for 6 years, scientists found that *any* kind and amount of exercise helped extend life. Pushing a lawn mower, climbing stairs, sweeping, walking the dog, even standing rather than sitting while talking on the phone. What works is simply calories burned, with those burning the most from these activities of daily living having a 69 percent lower risk of dying than those who burned the least.

You can even burn up to 350 calories a day just by fidgeting. Volunteers were fed 1,000 extra calories a day for 8 weeks (an amount that many of us consume regularly!). Some people gained 2 pounds, others as much as 16. The difference? How much they fiddled and fidgeted.

The chart on page 162 shows you the calories you'll burn per hour for a variety of activities. Please note these are just estimates—the exact amount of calories that you'll burn depends on your weight and physical fitness. And remember, moving for an hour may be difficult at first. Start with 15 to 20 minutes and make up the rest of your calorie burning by walking. To find out exactly how much you can burn on any activity, go to http://primusweb.com/cgi-bin/fpc/actcalc.pl.

"The dictionary is the only place that success comes before work. Hard work is the price we must pay for success. I think you can accomplish anything if you're willing to pay the price."
—*Vince Lombardi*

CALORIE BURN CHART
FOR ACTIVITIES OF 30-MINUTE DURATION

ACTIVITY	150-POUND WOMAN (CALORIES)	180-POUND MAN (CALORIES)
Gym Based		
Aerobics, high-impact	315	378
Aerobics, low impact	225	270
Elliptical trainer	324	389
Hatha yoga	113	135
Step aerobics (6" to 8" step)	383	459
Weight lifting, heavy	270	324
Weight lifting, light	135	162
Sports and Related		
Bicycling, 12 to 13.9 mph	360	432
Dancing (disco, ballroom, line, polka)	203	243
Golf, walking and pulling clubs	193	232
Horseback riding	180	216
Running 5.2 mph (11.5-minute mile)	405	486
Running up stairs	675	810
Skiing, cross country, 2.5 mph	315	378
Snowshoeing	360	432
Swimming, moderate, 50 yards/minute	360	432
Tennis, doubles, competitive	225	270
Walking, 3.5 mph (17-minute mile)	171	205
Outdoor Home Maintenance		
General gardening	180	216
Raking lawn	193	232
Shoveling snow with snow shovel	270	324
Home and Daily		
Child care (bathing, feeding, etc.)	135	162
Food shopping, with or without cart	103	124
General housecleaning	135	162
Playing with kids, moderate effort	180	216
Sleeping	40	49
Watching TV	45	54

ACTIVITY	150-POUND WOMAN (CALORIES)	180-POUND MAN (CALORIES)
Office Related		
Computer typing	68	81
Riding in a bus or vehicle to work	45	54
Standing, filing, light work	103	124
Occupational		
Bakery, moderate effort	180	216
Coaching sports	180	216
Horse grooming	270	324
Light office work	68	81
Nursing	135	162
Road construction	270	324
Sitting in class	81	97

5. Track It

Just like with calories in, people who do best in Muscle track calories burned. You can use a fancy computer program (although I've found that even athletes have a hard time keeping it up) or something as simple as a journal. The template in Appendix 2 is one way; find what works for you.

TO ENJOY:

If you scored a 2 to 4 on the endurance test, just take a quick look at the "To Survive" suggestions. If you feel you have them covered, you can start here.

1. Experience Walking Meditation

Let's say that you already have incorporated more vigorous cardio into your lifestyle. But you want a deeper mind-body-spirit experience. How about doing a walking meditation? Both Buddhism and Christianity have forms, but you can make it up as you go along. Find a peaceful place to walk. I love to walk where I can hear the sound of water—a babbling brook, a roaring river, or the ocean. It helps me find a core of tranquility. You can repeat a prayer or mantra to help you achieve this state of mind.

2. Be Daring

Now that you're more fit, how about doing something you've always considered daring? Hop on that trail bike. Get up on those water skis and fly over the waves. What about pole dancing, ladies? Strap on those rollerblades and glide into skatin' heaven. Always wanted to mountain climb? You haven't lived until you've seen the world from the top of a mountain—and it can be any size. One of my most successful patients was on an all-woman ice hockey team. She was the oldest and the boldest. Twenty pounds later, she was two dress sizes smaller and was a lean, mean, fearless fightin' machine.

TO CHALLENGE:

If you scored a 5 to 6 on the test, just take a quick look at the "To Survive" and "To Enjoy" tips. If you feel you have them covered, you can start here.

1. Cross-Train and Compete

Put your Fit to Live body to the test. Plan to train for a marathon, duathlon (run and bike), or triathlon (run, bike, swim). There are plenty of groups to take training classes with. If you

---

Voice of Success: Get a Buddy— It's Mutually Ensured Intimidation!

Bob and Saj Bartolo, in their sixties, have been running for over a quarter century

"We do triathlons and marathons for different reasons. Saj does it for the joy and interaction with others. Bob, so he doesn't have to be worried about becoming breathless going up stairs. We've done it so long and with such consistency that it's our lifestyle now. Almost every day, we do one or two things—a run, yoga, a bike ride. We're retired now, but even when we worked, we found a way to fit it in. After work, at lunch, on weekends. It helps to find something you love. Even when you love it, sometimes it's hard to do, so having an underlying passion makes it easier. For guys, it helps to have a goal—to do a 5-K in 3 months, for instance. We tell people to start really slow, like walking for 10 minutes, running for 20 seconds. It also helps to have a buddy system or join a running or biking club. Having someone rely on you to get out of bed on a rainy morning to meet them helps you—and them—keep your commitment. It's mutually ensured intimidation!"

don't want to compete right away, just cross-train to keep your whole body optimally challenged. People are often amazed to discover that they can bike or swim very well, but when asked to run, find they're calling 911 in 5 minutes. Or vice versa. That's because the body can be incredibly fit in one kind of endurance but not in others. To have maximum cardio fitness, give your body a variety of aerobic challenges. The more you mix it up, the less likely your body will overly adapt to one form and become stagnant.

2. Travel the World

Go global. Sign up for that 60- to 100-miles-per-day biking week in the south of France. Make plans now to hike up Machu Pichu in South America. What about doing the London marathon or biking across Northern Ireland? See the world in ways you never thought about before. You'll stay in magnificent shape and experience the thrill of learning about another culture.

3. Do a Group Challenge

There are now all kinds of events designed as relays. You get a team and each do a part—a marathon divided into 3-K or 6-K per person, two people doing half of a bike race, swim in a relay team for breast cancer. At the San Francisco marathon, there are even groups that run together in costumes. Or join a softball, basketball, or racquetball team. Just get out there, show up, have fun, and burn up that Toxic Belly Fat.

CHAPTER 9

Sculpting the Body

*"All we actually have is our body and its muscles that allow us
to be under our own power."*
—ALLEGRA KENT

Now it's time to concentrate on building and maintaining strong-enough muscles to prevent a fall, help you get up once you've fallen, or help carry someone else. These glorious muscles are your premium calorie burners as well. A pound of muscle burns three to five times the amount of calories compared with a pound of fat. Don't make the mistake of thinking that all you have to do is cardio to Cut your Toxic Belly Fat. You need strength training as well to get those calories off. Did you know that if you do regular strength training—lifting weights for 1 hour twice per week—you can eliminate Toxic Belly Fat three times faster than those people who are doing only cardio? For that matter, when you incorporate weight training along with your cardio, you can prevent Toxic Fat from accumulating in the first place. Finally, lifting those weights doubles your chance of keeping the Toxic Belly Fat off in the long term.

⇒Our Toxic Lifestyle⇐
Muscles? What Muscles?

"The health you enjoy is largely your choice."
—ABRAHAM LINCOLN

The farm and the factory was today's equivalent of a power-lifting gym. Building railroads or fences, mining, or cattle roping—it all required strength. So did women's work: chopping wood to cook with, churning, carrying heavy pails of water. Remember death by exhaustion? That was real.

These days, most of us are not as strong as we need to be. Sure, we can get by on a normal day, walking a few steps from the house to the car and back. But let's stress you for a minute. Have you got the reserves to lift your suitcase into the overhead bin of the airplane without killing yourself or your fellow passengers? Are you strong enough to push that wheelbarrow in your garden? A friend invites you to go rafting. Do you have the upper-body strength to be able to say yes? Your automatic garage door opener isn't working, and you have to manually pull it down. Can you?

What if your life depended upon your strength? Think back to the spider lady in Chapter 1. She faced the possibility of death or certainly disability if she had fallen down those steps instead of having the strength, at 63, to hold onto the branches and right herself. Because she was Fit to Live, when her comfort zone was replaced by a crisis, she had the reserves to save her life.

As a society, we haven't prioritized strength training. Only 20 percent of us are doing strength training twice a week, with women slightly trailing men. That means 80 percent of us are ignoring this crucial aspect of being Physically Fit to Live. If we don't get at it, we're going to be a culture of frail, fat folks with fractures. Here's why: The body was built for obsolescence after the age of 50. One of the ways it does that is by dropping muscle mass if you're not using it. Between 30 and 50, a sedentary woman can drop

"Obstacles don't have to stop you. If you run into a wall, don't turn around and give up. Figure out how to climb it, go through it, or work around it."
—*Michael Jordan*

Fascinating FAToid
Where Did I Put Those Keys?

Strength training, along with aerobics, keeps your mind sharp. It increases the amount of your gray matter (that's your neurons) in as little as 6 months and helps the brain plan, remember, and multitask better. And you're never too old to benefit. This research was done on elderly folks. **Bottom line:** Strength training helps you lift mental and physical weight.

between 5 and 10 pounds of muscle mass on average. And after the age of 50, this loss begins to accelerate, up to 6 pounds per decade through sheer disuse. As usual, men drop too, but will still have the metabolic advantage since they're starting with so much more.

Losing muscle mass is not good for you. First, your strength diminishes. But losing muscle decreases the flames in that calorie-burning furnace and increases your percentage of body fat. As a result, it's easier to pile on that Toxic Belly Fat, increasing your risk of diabetes, heart disease, and stroke threefold by changing how your body handles blood sugar and by altering the levels of fats in your blood.

No matter your age, if you do strength training, you not only reverse muscle loss, but actually build more. Even 80-year-olds who were once wheelchair- and walker-dependent have been shown to decrease fat mass and increase muscle mass through weight training.

Here's another reason to lift those weights. As we age, we also lose bone, which can lead to osteoporosis, a disorder that increases your risk of fractures. Weight-bearing exercise helps prevent osteoporosis two ways: by building bone and by slowing its loss. I've never seen women hop to it faster with weight training than when they are given the choice of either going on osteoporosis drugs with side effects like stomach upset, or lifting weights. Men, osteoporosis hits you too. We have the data to suggest that after the age of 70, it becomes a real problem.

One in 3 women and 1 in 12 men will suffer from osteoporosis at some point. Even if you don't have osteoporosis, if you fall—which happens a lot, especially for you happy campers over the age of 50—and are not strong, the likelihood of breaking something increases precipitously. But if you're strong, you decrease the odds of breaking a bone.

Women who are 45 and over were not raised in an era where women lifted weights. There's usually a bit of resistance to the idea. I'm thinking of a woman I met during one of

Fascinating FAToid

Get a Grip

Older men were tested for grip strength and then retested 7 years later. They had lost an average of 20 percent of their capacity. The older they were, the more they lost. **Bottom line:** You can't open a jar or hold scissors properly without grip strength, to name just two activities of daily living. Keep working your muscles, and you'll have the strength to live independently into your nineties or beyond.

my Peeke Week Retreats who was 60 years old and about 30 pounds overweight. Most of her weight was Toxic Belly Fat. She heard my seminar on strength training and came up to me afterward. "My husband told me that it's unladylike to lift weights," she confessed.

At first, I was shocked. But then I realized she came from a generation where ladies didn't do such things. And so did her husband. I asked her what else was holding her back. She said, "Well, I start sweating, and when I sweat, I mess up my hair and makeup, and I have to redo it, and it's uncomfortable, and I'm feeling some pains. . . . "

"Yes," I said. "That's your muscles awakening. You will feel a little bit of discomfort, but under the right supervision and guidance, you'll be fine."

Later, I spoke with her husband. "She's got to get this weight off because it's mostly in her belly. She has high blood pressure and is at high risk for heart disease. All the cardio in the world isn't going to get her there, at least no time soon."

He heard me loud and clear. I saw her a year later, and the first thing she did was whip up her sleeve and show me a very fine biceps. After showing off a normal-size waistline.

WATCH YOUR HIPS!

The most dangerous risk of osteoporosis? Hip fractures. Fifty percent of those who get a hip fracture can no longer live independently, and 20 percent die within 20 months. So start lifting today if you want to stay Alert and Vertical and independent into your golden years.

⇒Fit to Live⇐
Strong and Lean for Life

> "It is amazing how much crisper the general experience of life becomes when your body is given a chance to develop a little strength."
> —FRANK DUFF

The Fit to Live body is characterized by strength, by an optimal lean body mass (muscle) and minimized body fat. How do you do that? By sculpting your body to remove fat and increase muscle mass as much as your genetics allow and holding it there for a lifetime. You'll look and feel absolutely fabulous, create huge reserves of Body Dollars, and increase your chances of remaining Alert and Vertical as long as possible.

I began weight training over 25 years ago. A trainer at a very small club walked up to me one day when I was on a treadmill, touched my biceps, and said, "Did you ever think of weight training?"

I said, "I don't even know what that is."

I'd done years of ballet and aerobics. But no one had ever paid attention to my muscle. He took me over to the free weights area, and I lifted my first weight—a single-digit one, mind you. I woke up the next morning aching in places I didn't know I owned. However, the weirdest thing happened. I felt stronger mentally! I could feel my muscles as I moved. These little discomforts were making me aware of my body in a new way. I was hooked.

I'm guessing you'll love it as much as I do. The journey starts with my five Fit to Live principles.

THE FIVE FIT TO LIVE STRENGTH-TRAINING PRINCIPLES

1. You Have to Lift Weight to Remove Weight

Aerobic activity burns fuel. But weight training tells you how fast you'll burn it. Strength training both builds more muscle and increases the calorie-burning efficiency of the muscle you have. For each pound of trained muscle on your body, you can burn 35 to 50 calories of energy per day. Each pound of fat requires only 7 to 10 calories to maintain it. Quite a difference. When you lift weights, you are able to burn calories faster because you need more calories to feed those hungry muscle cells. That's why it's key to trimming that Toxic Belly Fat.

If I were going to look under your hood, I'd see muscles. What kind of shape are they in? Do you have enough of them? The more there are and the stronger they are, the faster you'll drop fat from your body because you become more efficient at burning calories.

Sit down in a stuffed chair. Can you get out without holding on to the arms? (You saw this in the test.) Guess what? You're squatting your own weight. Now, if you are obese—carrying at least 50 pounds more than you need—your leg muscles are incredibly strong. You are your own gym! All day long, you are power-lifting with your legs, whether you're walking, getting out of chairs, or climbing stairs. From the pelvis on down, you are really strong. (Which is why heavier people burn more calories when walking, because they're doing more work and their leg muscles are larger.) So you may find the lower-leg work at the end of this chapter easy to do but have a lot more trouble with the upper-body ones. What's important to understand here is no matter what your size, you can use your own weight to get strong—no barbells needed.

2. You Have the Right to Bare Arms and Bellies

Aren't you tired of "hide-it" clothes? Especially those that hide the upper body? It's depressing and mentally exhausting to wake up every day and have to spend time desperately choosing clothes that camouflage bat wings and bellies. You deserve to be able to

Fascinating FAToid
Want to Feel Good about Yourself?
Strength training actually boosts body image for men and women. When men and women did strength training 5 days a week for 12 weeks, they not only got stronger, removed fat, and added muscle, but the men felt good about themselves for doing the training. Women did too, but they also got a body image boost by the objective evidence of strength gains. **Bottom line:** Track your progress, ladies; evidence of your physical abilities will make you feel better about your body.

Fascinating FAToid

Make Friends with Your Personal Calorie Burners

Every pound of trained muscle (used every day) burns 35 to 50 calories. A pound of fat, on the other hand, burns only 7 to 10 calories. **Bottom line:** Fan those metabolic fires with hot, trained muscles.

open that closet door and whip through your wardrobe, grabbing that beautiful white blouse and tucking it into sexy jeans. Men, who needs to sweat BOB (belly over belt) anymore? How about wearing a belt that's actually even with your belly button? You can achieve this glorious body baring the fastest by emphasizing your upper-body workout.

3. Your Core Is Key

Remember, we've been talking about staying Alert and Vertical for as long as possible? Building muscle is about vertical. Because of our lack of physical fitness, we have a collapsing core (abdomen). That's not a good thing. To have a nice strong, tall back with excellent posture, you've got to be strong at your core. This gets more important as you get older because your body has a natural tendency to shrink.

Core strength training is absolutely essential to shedding Toxic Belly Fat. First, you become more aware of your abdomen. This mental awareness helps you stay focused on your goal—to eliminate the excess inner abdominal fat and achieve your goal of a waist

Voice of Success: From Weight to Whistles

Jan Swarthout, forties, removed 75 pounds of body fat

"My trainer recently did my measurements, and I'm at 18 percent body fat. I was featured in the gym newsletter. People out of nowhere come up to me, grab my hand, and say job well done. I am so thrilled! It was really hard work but worth it. Lifting weights gives the toning and definition your body needs, while tightening up the loose skin. It was key to removing fat, as well as cardio and eating right. I now wear a size 6 or 8. I bought my first tankini! I haven't worn a bathing suit for 10 years. Guys whistle at me if I am running or exercising outside. What FUN!"

that is less than 35 inches for women and less than 40 inches for men. Core training also builds a stronger calorie-burning furnace when you build more muscle. Remember, you're not just building abdominal muscles; you're also building back muscles. This is a tremendous win/win in the challenge to shed those Toxic Belly Fat pounds.

Why else does posture matter? Well, just for grins, hunch over like the hunchback of Notre Dame. Now try to take a deep breath. You can't because your diaphragm's up in your neck somewhere!

Now straighten up, just like the teacher ordered when we were kids in school. Throw those shoulders back! Now you've got that nice posture, which, by the way, will become so much easier and natural as your strength increases. Take a deep breath. Hear that clank? That was your diaphragm hitting the floor. Which means you can breathe deeply, which makes it easier and more efficient for you to walk, run, bike, swim, go up the stairs. And save your life as well.

Okay, let's go back to slouch position. Look down at your belly. Skinny or obese, what happens? Your belly sticks out! Now go back to the beautiful straight posture. Now look at your belly. It flattens out! This works for everyone, no matter what size your belly is— the better the posture, the flatter your abdomen.

Having a strong core is not only for breathing well, but it also is key to all kinds of daily activities like sitting down, picking things up, carrying groceries, even walking. The abs and the back work together as a team—the stronger the abs, the stronger the back. And vice versa. That's why the routine at the end of the chapter works both.

SCULPTING SECRETS

1. Do reps carefully, using good form to avoid injuring joints.
2. When you lift, aim to keep increasing the intensity by exercising each muscle thoroughly and gradually increasing the weights.
3. Wear weight-lifting gloves for a more secure grip and wrist straps to stabilize your wrist when lifting heavier weights.
4. If you're using machines at the gym, make sure they are adjusted to your height. Have a trainer help you get the right settings and then write them down on a card so you can reproduce them on your own.

SHOULD YOU GET A TRAINER?

My program is designed to get you lean and strong safely and swiftly. But having a trainer has been shown to help people achieve better results by increasing intensity and consistency. If you do get one, be sure he or she is accredited by an organization like the American College of Sports Medicine or the National Strength and Conditioning Association. You can also get individual and group support at the Muscle section of my Web site, which also offers a list of questions to ask a potential trainer.

---

4. Do It Twice a Week—with Vitamin I: Intensity!

Do not lift weights every day. Do not even lift weights four times a week. All you need to do is infuse your workout with vitamin I—lift weight with intensity twice a week for about 30 minutes. The workout I give at the end of the chapter fits the bill. Notice I said "with intensity"—if you're just going through the motions, you won't get the results you want. Really work those muscles!

First, concentrate on your form. Form is everything in weight training. To achieve this, have a fitness professional shows you appropriate form. Study the models in this book as they demonstrate each exercise. As you begin a specific exercise move, realize that muscle is stimulated to grow when it is working the hardest. In a biceps curl, it's the journey up that's the toughest. Count it out. A count of four as you contract to get up all the way, and a count of three to release and come down. If you run through them too quickly, you'll not only injure yourself, but you won't get the optimal muscle training, toning, and definition you want.

As you begin, get that patience into play. Women, it will take you about 6 weeks to build that pound of muscle. Men, probably closer to 4 weeks.

The exercises I show at the end of the chapter can all be done at home. The ones at the Survival level are done using your own weight, so you don't need special equipment. At the Enjoy and Challenge levels, I've given exercises using resistance bands, dumbbells, and fitness balls, which you can buy at any sporting goods store.

> "I think exercise is the fountain of youth. If it were a pill, everyone would be taking it."
> —*Rita Redberg, MD*

5. Pen Your Progress

When you begin to weight train, there seems to be a dizzying array of exercises. This is particularly true for women who may never have done any weight training before. So, we've made it easy. The chart in Appendix 2 helps you track your progress. There's also a chart to pen your progress with body comp, girth, and bone density.

As you learned in the Mouth section, you need to keep track of your body comp. Either have an experienced fitness professional do it, or buy one of those body-fat scales we talked about earlier.

⇒Fit to Live Essentials⇐

Using your score from the strength test, you'll continue to build your individual program with the tips below. As in previous chapters, you'll begin according to your current level. Make certain you have mastered your level for that particular exercise before advancing to the next. For instance, you may find that your biceps are at the Challenge level but your triceps are struggling at the Survive level. That's fine. You're supposed to mix it up, because everyone has a variety of physical strengths and weaknesses. The goal is to move from Survive to Enjoy. Then, strive to push yourself further by trying the Challenge level if you feel you've mastered that Enjoy level exercise.

I have tried to make this a gymless experience so that these exercises are more accessible to everyone. I want you to see that your own living environment can provide great opportunities to get Fit to Live. You'll use a sturdy chair, a simple workout mat, a fitness ball, and a simple set of single hand dumbbells (for women from 3 to 15 pounds, for men from

Fascinating FATroid
This Is Smokin' News!

Smokers who combine exercise with nicotine gum or transdermal patches are more likely to quit than those who rely on nicotine-replacement therapy alone. And those who exercised were more likely to reduce their cigarette smoking if they did not quit. They also scored better on several tests measuring respiratory health. **Bottom line:** Lifting and walking are your best help to get off those cigarettes.

> "Physical fitness is not only one of the most important keys to a healthy body, it is the basis of dynamic and creative intellectual activity."
>
> —*John F. Kennedy*

5 to 30 pounds). Dedicate a small area in the house for doing these exercises. Wear comfortable clothing. Walking sneakers and socks work great. I wear a loose pair of shorts and a T-shirt, both of which have to be a million years old. But hey, it's your house, and this isn't a fashion show. We're here to buckle down and get Fit to Live!

You will do your strength training workout twice a week. Each session will be 30 minutes long. After each set of repetitions, rest for 5 to 10 seconds and then continue. If you do your twice-a-week training regularly, you will notice a significant increase in strength over the course of the first 6 weeks. As you become more Fit to Live, it will become easier to increase the intensity for each exercise. As you increase intensity, your strength and endurance increase as well.

TO SURVIVE:

If you received a score of 0 to 4 on the strength test, focus your energy here first. Once you've mastered these, feel free to move up to the program in "To Enjoy." Do the exercise slowly and precisely to get the most benefit. Your goal is to do each exercise 10 times (repetitions or reps) for three sets. To start, just try one or two reps and see how you feel. If it's been a while since you've exercised, you'll feel some burning in the quadriceps or thigh muscles. As you train more regularly, most of this will go away. For this level, you'll need a chair—that's it!

DON'T FORGET YOUR BONES!

The measurement of your Toxic Belly Fat is important, but you also need to know your bone density. Women, get a bone density baseline at age 40 to 45 and then monitor it depending on what you find out. Do you have a family history of osteoporosis or osteopenia? Hop on it now. Don't wait until you're 50. Men, I would recommend starting to measure at around 60.

Chair Squat

Sit in a firm-backed chair with your feet shoulder-width apart, toes pointing straight forward, and arms crossed across your chest.

Take a deep breath and as you let the air out, get up from the chair by extending your knees. Arms should remain across your chest. Keep your abdominal muscles tucked in with your belly button toward the spine. Return to the starting position by bending your knees. Repeat 10 times.

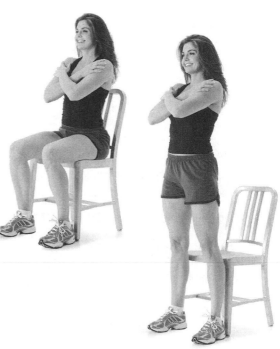

Lateral Side Step

Stand with your feet shoulder-width apart, toes pointing straight forward, hands at the waist, and knees slightly bent. Take a lateral step to the right, maintaining your bent knees and your erect posture. Switch sides. Repeat 10 times.

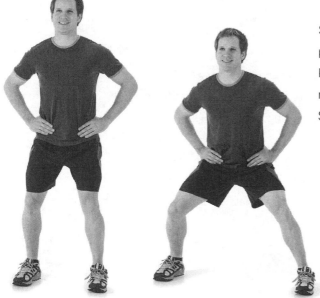

↘ Wall Pushup

From a standing position, face a flat wall about an arm's length away. Feet should be shoulder-width apart, toes facing straight forward. Place both hands at chest level against the wall.

Bend your elbows toward the wall, maintaining an erect posture with your abdominal muscles tucked in. Return to the starting position by extending your elbows. Repeat 10 times.

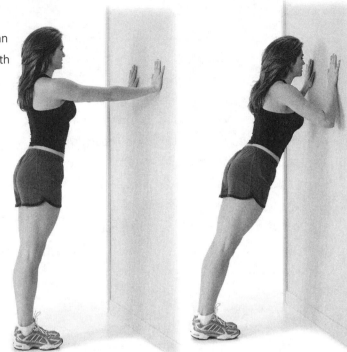

Prone Back Extension ↙

Lie flat on your stomach, arms by your side, forehead touching the mat. Take a deep breath prior to movement.

As you let the air out, lift your chest off the mat, maintaining a long neck by keeping your face toward the mat. Return to the starting position. Repeat 10 times.

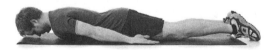

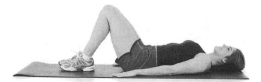

Supine Bent-Knee Pelvic Tilt

Lie flat on your back, knees bent, feet hip-width apart, toes facing straight forward, arms by your side, and hands flat against the floor.

Take a deep breath and tilt your pelvis, bringing your hip bones toward your ribs. Gently press your palms against the floor. During your exhale, return to the starting position. Repeat 10 times.

TO ENJOY:

If you scored a 5 to 9 on the strength test, just take a quick look at the "To Survive" exercises. I would recommend that you run through them and make certain you are comfortable with each exercise. Remember, you may find that you are at the Survive level for some of the exercises and the Enjoy or even Challenge level for others. You are going to customize your program to fit your individual needs. If you feel you're fine with the Survive level, then let's start right into the Enjoy exercises.

Body Squat—Unassisted

From a standing position, place your feet shoulder-width apart, with your hands at your waist.

Inhale and squat down as if you were sitting on a chair. Keep your chest erect, with your knees over your toes as you descend. Hold the position for a count of five. Exhale as you return to the starting position. Perform two sets of 10 repetitions each.

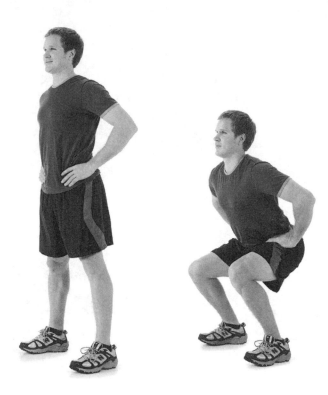

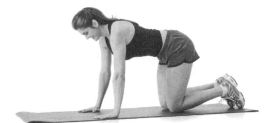

Bent-Knee Pushup

Start on your hands and knees, maintaining a flat back, with your hands on the floor directly under each shoulder.

Inhale as you bend your elbows as if you were going to touch the floor with your nose. Stop at approximately a 90-degree angle, with your elbows in line with your shoulders. Exhale and return to the starting position. Perform one or two sets of 10 repetitions.

Supine Bent-Knee Pelvic Tilt/ Bridges with One Leg Extended

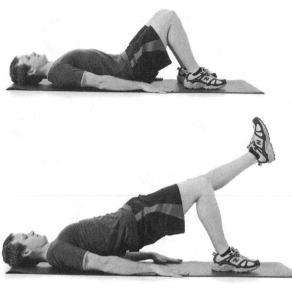

Lie flat on your back with your knees bent, feet hip-width apart, toes facing straight forward, arms by your side, and hands flat against the floor.

Take a deep breath and tilt your pelvis, bringing your hip bones toward your ribs. Lift your buttocks off the floor. Gently press the palms of your hands against the floor. Hold the position and extend one leg forward, pressing your knees together. During your exhale, return to the starting position. Switch legs. Repeat five times with each leg.

TO CHALLENGE:

If you scored a 10 to 14 on the strength test, just take a quick look at the "To Survive" and "To Enjoy" exercises. Go ahead and try as many of them as you wish. Again, you may find that although your overall score was high, there may be specific problem areas for you. Maybe your leg muscles are great but your biceps aren't. Remember, this is all about customizing a program that honors your unique physical needs. At the Challenge level, we're ramping up the difficulty to meet the needs of men and women who have passed the Survive and Enjoy levels and want to challenge themselves further. You'll need a set of dumbbells and a fitness ball. Men can start with 8- to 10-pound dumbbells and women 3 to 8 pounds. Each person needs to experiment and see what feels right. It's always wise to start light; it reduces the risk of injury. You want to feel a moderate burn or strain from the exercise, but no pain. You will move up when you can perform the exercise with no perception of strain whatsoever. Then you increase and gradually work your way up by 1- to 2-pound increments with the goal of feeling that moderate muscular strain of a challenging exercise.

Body Squat with Biceps Curl

From a standing position, place your feet shoulder-width apart and hold dumbbells down at your sides.

Squat down as if you were sitting on a chair and curl your arms. Keep your chest erect, knees over your toes as you descend. Return to the starting position and lower the dumbbells. Inhale as you descend and exhale as you ascend. Perform two sets of 10 repetitions each.

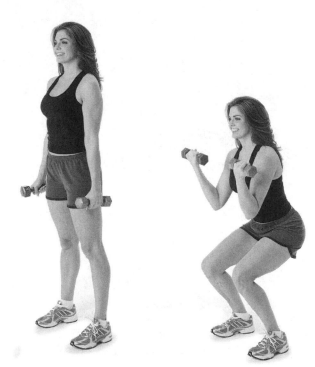

Floor Pushup

Start in a plank position, as pictured.

Bend your elbows, lowering your entire body midway toward the floor. Return to the starting position by extending elbows. Maintain an erect posture. Keep abdominal muscles tight. Perform one set of 10 repetitions.

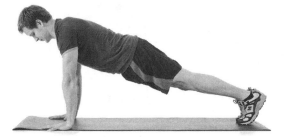

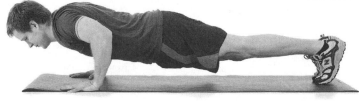

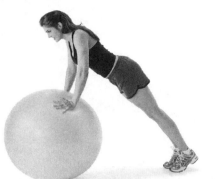

Ball Pushup

Place your hands on the ball.

Bend the elbows, bringing the whole body midway toward the floor. Return to the starting position by extending your elbows. Maintain an erect posture. Keep abdominal muscles tight.

Ball Trunk Flexion

Sit on the ball with your feet planted firmly on the floor.

Walk your feet forward until your midback rests on the ball. Support your head with your hands. Curl your trunk, lifting your upper back off the ball, and return to the starting position. Do one set of 10 repetitions.

CHAPTER 10

Stretching and Balancing the Body

"Take care of your body. It's the only place you have to live."
—*JIM ROHN*

I asked you to be mentally flexible in the Mind section, right? In this chapter, we'll explore why you need to be physically flexible. If you don't, eventually you will have very limited range of motion in your joints. As you age, you might even become unable to bend over to pick something off the floor or twist to reach for something.

Another aspect of Muscle that's equally important but often overlooked is your balance. We must do balance exercises, because our sense of balance deteriorates as we age. And balance is one of the keys to walking, people! With the simple exercises you'll learn to do here, you'll automatically have the flexibility and balance basics covered. You'll release pent-up stress and feel more secure, knowing your body is Fit to Live to survive and enjoy your life—and save it, too, if need be!

⇒Our Toxic Lifestyle⇐
Overstressed and Understretched

"You have got to take care of the most important person in the world, YOU! For many of these guys, the only thing they think about is making money and they forget about their body. Without their body, they are nothing."
—JACK LALANNE

In the East, people have understood the need for flexibility and balance for thousands of years. Yoga in India, tai chi and chi gong in China, Thai massage in Thailand. All these mind/body/spirit practices allowed practitioners to stay supple and balanced into great old age. In the West, we've traditionally not paid specific attention to these key markers of fitness. Nor did we need to, not at least in centuries past, because we maintained our balance and flexibility by working for our survival. Whether we were hunters and gatherers or on the farm or in factories, we had many occasions each day to twist, stretch, reach, bend, and balance. Most of us didn't live very long, so we didn't have to worry about these consequences of aging.

As we began to live longer and work our bodies less, we began to experience what we thought of as symptoms of old age—lack of flexibility and loss of balance among them. These are not automatic consequences of the passing years; they are the results of disuse.

Fascinating FAToid
A Different Kind of Nursing Home Insurance

By keeping balance good, people over age 65 reduce the risk of falling, which can result in death, head injuries, and bone fractures, as well as being admitted to a nursing home for a year or longer. Think it's not likely? More than one-third of adults over 65 fall each year, and more than 1.8 million seniors were treated in emergency rooms for fall-related injuries in 2003. And why do people fall? Lack of balance. **Bottom line:** Balance exercises keep you out of the hospital and help you stay independent.

> "Safeguard the health both
> of body and soul."
> —*Cleobulus*

But this isn't just an aging problem. As a result of our tremendous lack of flexibility, there's a whole crowd of younger people out there right now who can't perform the tasks of daily living. They can't put their shoes on, for instance, because they're too big and inflexible to bend over far enough. In fact, an entire line of products has been created for people who lack flexibility. I'm not talking about supporting people who are old and frail. I'm talking about people who should be able to tie their shoes. There are now Web sites offering sock installers and leg lifters, longer shower hoses and lotion applicators, large body sponges on handles for reaching feet. All because people can't bend and reach, mostly because of Toxic Fat.

Young or old, to stay balanced, we have to balance. To stay flexible, we have to stretch. We've got to bank those Body Dollars so we'll have the reserve we need. How come? To avoid the one thing that we dread so much—falling. When you fall at any age, and you lack flexibility and balance, then you may not just break bones or hit your head, but you could end up in the hospital and pick up some infection. Then it's game over.

As far as balance goes, there are sensors in our ears that help with this important ability. As we age, they don't work as well unless we keep using them. Because we're not staying active enough, by age 75, loss of balance is one of the most common reasons people go to the doctor.

Inactivity causes muscles, tendons, and ligaments to shorten. That's true for us all. But especially after the age of 40, your ligaments get drier. It's a natural part of the aging process. If you don't stay consistent with stretching, you won't be greasing your ligaments enough to keep them supple. But it's not only to stay supple when we're old. Stretching's also been found to help us:

o Keep our balance
o Have better posture
o Improve circulation
o Relieve stress
o Reduce back and arthritis pain

We used to believe that stretching before exercise decreases injuries, but research has disproven that. What we do know is that stretching increases our "stretch tolerance,"

Fascinating FAToid

Back and Knee Pain Alert

Do you have a "bad" back or knees? More than 80 percent of us do, at some point. Up to 60 percent of those with such problems are suffering from tight hamstrings and hips due to a lack of flexibility. **Bottom line:** Stretching helps give us back more ability to move our bodies and enjoy life.

meaning we feel less pain when the same force is applied to the muscle. So it allows us to work our bodies more without experiencing pain.

The bottom line on flexibility and balance: It's a big "use it or lose it" thing. And because so many of us have ignored this aspect of being Physically Fit to Live, we've really lost it. Time once again to create those reserves so that you'll have the wonderful, painless range of motion in the Body Dollar bank for as long as you need!

⇨ Fit to Live ⇦

Head, Shoulders, Knees, and Toes

"A problem not anticipated is a problem . . . a problem anticipated is an opportunity!
—JOHN C. MAXWELL

As baby boomers hit their fifties and sixties, those who are Fit to Live are getting the message about flexibility and balance. That's one of the reasons for the popularity of yoga, tai chi, chi gong, and yogalates (a combo of Pilates and yoga), as well as balance training being named one of the hottest trends in fitness. All these approaches not only help you develop greater flexibility and balance, they also strengthen your core (the abdominals and lower back muscles you learned about in Chapter 9). A strong core helps you be able to bend over without falling on the dog or reach up to get something out of a cabinet without toppling over.

Like the other Muscle elements, there's a slew of conflicting advice. I've distilled it down. You'll be amazed at how simple it can be.

THE FIVE FIT TO LIVE FLEXIBILITY AND BALANCE PRINCIPLES

1. Whether You Have a Gen X or Y, a Primer, or a Boomer Body, Start Flexing Now

Regardless what your age is, start stretching and balancing right now. Build a strong foundation so you'll be able to roll right through all your years without so much of the stiffness and pain of the sedentary man or woman. Younger people may think this issue is something you worry about when you pass 40 or 50.

Wrong. If you want to have fun with any form of recreation—organized sports, fun vacations, and adventure trips—then better balance and flexibility will help you optimize the experience. You cannot take up running or tennis without stretching. You need it to avoid injury and achieve a winning performance. Heck, stretching helps you survive hours of sedentary desk work as you navigate school and new careers. For that matter, this cer-

---

Voice of Success: "My Husband Calls Me a Gym Rat."

Shirley Abbott Clark removed 42 pounds, 38 of them fat, and is still going down

"I like to say I walked my butt off one step at a time. I have a very slow metabolism and have to do an hour a day 5 days a week. My husband calls me a gym rat. Recently, I've had a lot of injuries—a cyst on my ankle, broken toe, sprained ankle. But that's life. It's like sales. When you get a no, you have to accept it and turn it into a winning situation. With these injuries, stretching has become more important. Before, I would go do something on a weekend and then be tight and not do anything for 6 months. Now, I need to stay loose to keep my activity up. When I stretch right, it hurts at first. I've learned to breathe into it and then I loosen. I was having back pain, which turned out to be connected to my hamstrings. Stretching took care of that. What I'm really doing is turning back the clock. I look and feel a lot better than I did 10 years ago. But you have to be willing to do the work. I do it because I'm not going back to the way I used to feel."

tainly applies to the last trimester of preg- nancy, as you try to stay vertical with baby on board. And obviously, the more you practice stretching and balance work now, the easier your transition through the second half of your life. This is another non-negotiable prescription I'm giving you here. Integrate your balance and flexibility exercises into your daily routine.

> "A sound mind in a sound body is a short but full description of a happy state in this world."
>
> —*John Locke*

2. It Takes Only 5 Minutes after Your Daily Cardio

Why so little time? A daily stretch of each muscle group can increase range of motion in as little as 30 seconds. But in general, say experts, you won't get any further benefit from 60 seconds or from doing it more than once for 30 seconds. How's that for minimum effort required? The same applies for the balance exercises.

Why do these after cardio? Because then one reminds you of the other. Some folks also say that it's easier to do without hurting yourself once your muscles have been warmed up. A walk will accomplish that goal quite easily. If you get busy and it's tricky to even get your cardio in, don't worry. Try to hit the stretching and balance work no less than three times a week and strive for five.

3. Gentle, People!

When you stretch, your muscle fiber is pulled out to its full length and then the connective tissue is also pulled. When you hold it in that stretched out position, your body's stretch reflex is triggered, meaning it sends a signal to contract. As you hold it in that position, the stretch reflex stops signaling, and it relaxes at the longer length.

If you haven't stretched in a long time (or ever), don't expect to be a yoga expert on day one. You can rip and tear your muscles and ligaments if you stretch too violently. Ouch! Also, don't bounce. That also increases the risk of tearing a ligament or something. And when I say gentle, I mean it. Ligaments can tear when stretched only 6 percent more than their normal length. That's not very much.

To do it without hurting yourself, move slowly and carefully into position. Stretch until you feel a slight pulling but no pain. Breathe normally. As you hold, the muscle will relax, and you may be able to increase the stretch a bit more until you feel pulling again. Move slowly out. No quick moves or jerking. Do the same stretch on the other side.

4. Aim for Your Toes, Even if You Never Get There

You'll quickly discover that you're more flexible in some joints than others and perhaps more on one side than the other. That's okay. What you want to do is to help create the best range of motion you can, given your particular body. In general, the older you are, the longer it will take you to become more flexible. It's also influenced by previous injuries and how much muscle mass and extra body fat you have. Be curious about your abilities: Can I be more flexible today than yesterday? Can I get my head to my knee today?

You'll likely notice the same thing about balance. One side may be much easier than the other. Again, see how much you can challenge yourself: Can I stand on one leg without falling over longer today? Remember—start where you are and seek progress, not perfection!

5. It's Mini-Chill Time

One of the great things about doing flexibility and balance exercises is that it gives you a chance to take a mini-chill. You have to go slowly and listen to your body. So it's great for reducing stress. Plus, it just plain feels good—and we all can use more of that! If you're at the Enjoy or Challenge level, in addition to the workout I give here, consider yoga or one of the martial arts that allow you to practice mind and body. One of the most amazing people I've ever met was a woman who started tai chi at the age of 60. You should see her hold that crane pose at 70. She proves it's never too late.

Fascinating FAToid

Did You Know That . . . ?

People are more flexible in the afternoon than the morning (2:30 to 4 p.m. being the most flexible time), in warmer temperatures, and, say some experts, if they drink enough water. Women tend to be more flexible than men, and kids who haven't hit puberty are more so than adults. If you've got a lot of scarred muscle tissue, it will never be as flexible as unscarred tissue. **Bottom line:** Whatever your situation, just stay consistent and optimize that fantastic flexibility.

⇒Fit to Live Essentials⇐

Using your score from the third part of the "Are You Physically Fit to Live?" test, you'll continue to build your individual program with the exercises below. As in previous chapters, you'll begin according to your current level. If you're at the Enjoy level, just do the Survive exercises once to convince yourself that you can do them all. Then move on and strive to master the Enjoy exercises. Once that is accomplished, move onto the Challenge level.

Like the Strength and Core exercises in Chapter 9, don't be surprised if you find your skills cover more than one level. That's fine. You're going to customize your workout to fit your particular physical strengths and weaknesses.

These are gymless workouts. All you need is a comfortable place in your home and preferably a flat, uncarpeted floor to maximize balance. Wear comfortable clothing. Walking sneakers and socks work great. You will do your stretching and balance training along with your endurance workout. Each session will be anywhere from 5 to 10 minutes in duration. If you do your weekly stretching and balance training regularly, you will notice a significant increase in both over the course of the first 6 weeks. As you become more trained and have mastered the exercises at your level, feel free to advance to the next level. Once you've reached the Challenge level, just keep practicing the exercises as an integral part of your overall Fit to Live workout.

TO SURVIVE:

If you received a score of 0 to 4 on the flexibility and balance test, focus your energy here first. Once you've mastered these, feel free to move up to the exercises in "To Enjoy." Do these stretches after your calorie-burning workout, when you're all loose and warm.

FIT TO LIVE MUSCLE PLAN AT A GLANCE

DAY 1	DAY 2	DAY 3	DAY 4	DAY 5	DAY 6	DAY 7
Endurance/ Burn 300– 400 calories	Endurance/ Burn 300– 400 calories	Endurance/ Burn 300– 400 calories	Endurance/ Burn 300– 400 calories	Endurance/ Burn 300– 400 calories	Endurance/ Burn 300– 400 calories	Endurance/ Burn 300– 400 calories
Stretch / Balance 5 minutes	Stretch/ Balance 5 minutes	Stretch/ Balance 5 minutes	Stretch/ Balance 5 minutes	Stretch/ Balance 5 minutes	Stretch/ Balance 5 minutes	Stretch/ Balance 5 minutes
		Strength/ Core train 35 minutes		Strength/ Core train 35 minutes		

Hamstring Stretch

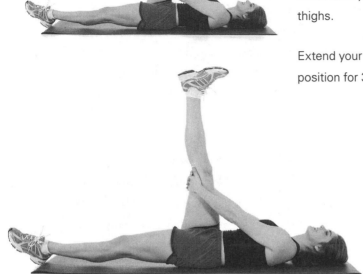

Lie flat on your back, and pull one knee toward your chest with your hands gently wrapped around your thighs.

Extend your leg toward the ceiling. Hold the position for 30 seconds. Switch sides.

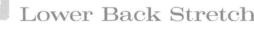 # Lower Back Stretch

Lie facedown on the floor, elbows bent, with palm facing down.

Gently press your hands against the floor while lifting your chest. Keep your hips against the floor. Hold the position for 30 seconds. Repeat two times.

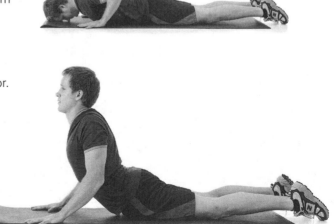

Calf Stretch

Stand facing a wall about 2 feet away. Place one foot closer to the wall, and place arms on wall at shoulder height.

Bend your front knee, while leaning the torso against the wall. Keep your back knee extended. Hold the position for 30 seconds. Switch sides.

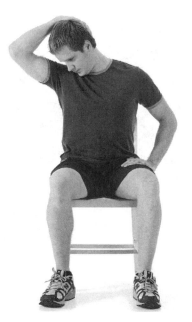

Neck Stretch

Seated on a chair, turn your head to the right, while gently pressing the back of your head with right hand, eyes pointing toward right shoulder. Hold the position for 30 seconds. Switch sides.

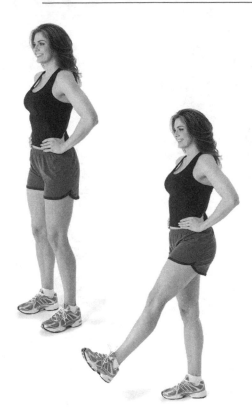

One-Leg Stance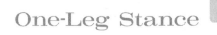

Stand with your feet shoulder-width apart and hands on your waist.

Raise one foot off the ground and balance for 5 seconds (maintaining balance and good posture). Switch sides. Repeat five times each side.

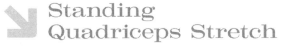# Standing Quadriceps Stretch

Stand with feet pointing straight forward, with your hands on your waist.

Bend one knee, bringing the foot toward the buttocks. Hold the position for 5 to 10 seconds. Switch sides.

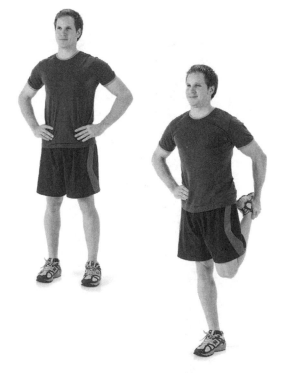

TO ENJOY:

If you scored a 5 to 9 on the flexibility and balance test, just take a quick look at the "To Survive" suggestions. If you feel you have them covered, you can start here. I would recommend that you run through them anyway and make certain you are comfortable with each exercise. Remember, you may find that you are at the Survive level for some of the exercises and Enjoy or even Challenge for others. You are going to customize your program to fit your individual needs. If you feel you're fine with the Survive level, then start right in to the Enjoy exercises.

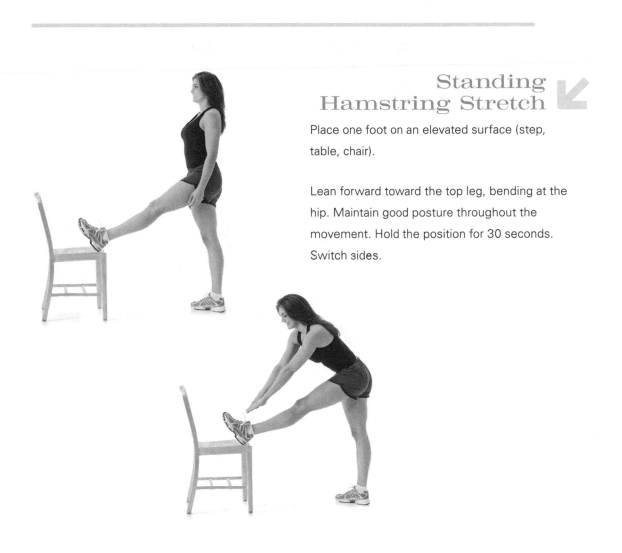

Standing Hamstring Stretch

Place one foot on an elevated surface (step, table, chair).

Lean forward toward the top leg, bending at the hip. Maintain good posture throughout the movement. Hold the position for 30 seconds. Switch sides.

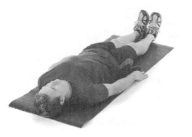

Piriformis Stretch

Lie flat on your back with legs extended.

Pull one knee toward your opposite shoulder using your opposite hand. Hold the position for 30 seconds. Switch sides.

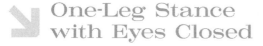

One-Leg Stance with Eyes Closed

Stand with your feet pointing straight forward.

Keeping your eyes closed, lift one foot off the floor with arms reaching forward. Hold the position for 5 to 10 seconds. Switch sides.

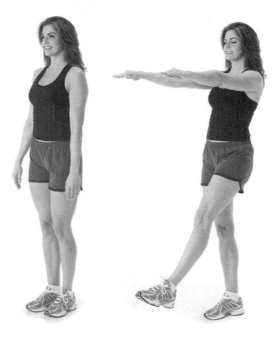

TO CHALLENGE:

If you scored a 10 to 14 on the flexibility and balance test, just take a quick look at the "To Survive" and "To Enjoy" suggestions. If you feel you have them covered, you can start here. Again, I would recommend you just do the Survive and Enjoy exercises once and make certain you have indeed mastered them before moving into the Challenge level. Some of the Enjoy folks are going to push themselves to try one or more Challenge exercises and strive to master them as they work on their other Enjoy exercises. That's perfectly fine. I noted before that your physical fitness may span several levels. You may simply be more limber than balanced, or vice versa. You have plenty of exercises to work with to experiment and customize your workout.

You'll know you've mastered the exercise when you can perform and repeat it without falling (balance) and when you can stretch without pain. Be patient. Never yank your arms or legs as you perform the exercises. You will feel some mild to moderate burn and discomfort as you stretch, but you should never feel pain. Both stretching and balance take at least 6 weeks of regular workouts to show significant improvement.

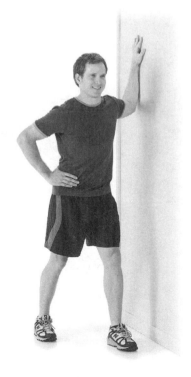

Standing Chest Stretch

Stand with one side facing a wall, one foot a shoulder's width in front of the other. Bend your arm 90 degrees, and place your elbow and forearm flat against the wall.

Gently press the inside forearm against the wall while bringing the chest slightly forward. Hold the position for 30 seconds. Switch sides.

Hip Stretch

Bend your knee and bring one leg over to the side, while keeping your shoulders flat on the floor. Hold the position for 30 seconds. Switch sides.

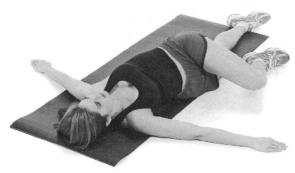

Squat and Jump

From a squatting position, jump and reach your arms toward the ceiling.

Land with your knees bent, keeping good form throughout. Repeat five times.

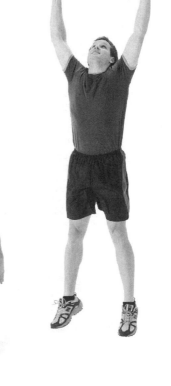

PART 4

Money: Are You Financially Fit to Live?

"The closer you are to your money, the better off you'll be."
—JASON FRIED

This section addresses the question, Am I Financially Fit to Live? To Survive, to Enjoy, to Challenge—and to save my life?

You're probably wondering why a doctor is writing about Financial Fitness. Well, in a nutshell, if you can't score a pair of sneakers, you ain't takin' a walk. I don't mean triple-digit fancy-shmancy sneakers hawked by some hip-hop star. I'm talking about a decent pair of shoes. Being Fit to Live isn't just about trekking off to the gym. You've got to pay for the gym. Got the $15 for your weekly Weight Watchers meeting? Or the money to pay for that healthy food?

If the goal is to live long and live well, and to avoid the Toxic Belly Fat problem, the newsflash is—wipe the shock off your face—you have to *pay* for this.

The next step in your Fit to Live journey is to be Financially Fit.

Of all the stresses in life, financial stress is one of the main reasons people fall off the healthy-living wagon. Overwhelmed with nightmares of becoming homeless and bankrupt, our last concern is "Gosh, did I eat enough fruits and vegetables today?" So many of my patients tell me that it was during times of financial distress that they fell into health-destructive habits to anesthetize the pain. We don't want to get into this position. We want to be able to have the money reserves to weather whatever financial storm erupts in our lives and still maintain our healthy lifestyle.

I rant and rave about making sure you see your primary-care practitioner for regular checkups and screenings. But you need the health insurance, deductibles, and co-payments to pay for this. I also tell you that you deserve to be Alert and Vertical for as long as you can. Note the word *long*. Do you have any idea how much it costs to live after age 50? Suddenly you're looking at another potentially 30 to 50 years of life, and most of us won't be working for a chunk of that.

The bottom line is that you need the Bank Dollars to optimize your Body Dollars, and vice versa. That, my friends, is why Health and Wealth management are so inextricably related. I worked with a team of financial experts to develop a plan to help you make the Bank Dollar/Body Dollar connection so you can become Fit to Live. In this section, you'll learn how to Cut the Bank Dollar debt. You'll stop wearing your nest egg as Toxic Belly Fat and invest it instead for your future.

To begin, find out your Financially Fit to Live level:

1. When it comes to credit cards, you:
   a. Charge only what you can pay off in full each month.
   b. Charge beyond your means so you can make only minimum payments, and then stress out over how you'll ever pay off the balances or ignore what the total is.
   c. Make payment in full online before the due date to eliminate interest payments.

2. Stress over money:
   a. Is a once-in-a-while kind of thing. You have a budget and some planning done, so only those unusual events, like a job loss, a hurricane, and illness or a market crash may create stress. In those cases, you get a bit stressed-out but consult your financial advisor for a plan adjustment.
   b. Causes you to overeat, drink, fight with a relative, stay awake at night, or fuel other habits that are ultimately bad for you.
   c. Doesn't happen. The war chest has been built, and you are ready to help those less fortunate than you.

3. When it comes time for retirement, you:

   a. Are not thinking about it yet. You are too busy thinking about meeting the financial demands of today.

   b. Expect to retire on a combination of Social Security, working a part-time job in retirement, and also some company-sponsored benefits. Maybe you have the benefits from your spouse as well.

   c. Are on track for saving enough to cover your income needs as well as your medical expenses in retirement. You are planning a new career living your dream while you are still healthy enough to do so.

4. If you were unable to take care of yourself due to health reasons, you:

   a. Would be forced to move in with relatives, and they would figure it out.

   b. Would probably go into a nursing care facility of some kind.

   c. Would use your savings and long-term-care insurance benefits to hire a caregiver in your own home.

5. What would your family do if you were to pass away unexpectedly?

   a. They would be in trouble. Your income is very important to sustaining the household.

   b. Your life insurance policy is enough to cover the gap in income and your services to the household, based on a thorough needs analysis.

   c. You have some life insurance through work. They would use that to make ends meet.

6. If your spouse or partner left, you would:

   a. Not know what to do.

   b. Have to get a better paying job right away.

   c. Have earned enough money on your own to support a decent lifestyle.

7. When it comes to retirement, which song title most reflects your attitude?

   a. "Sweet Dreams (Are Made of This)" by the Eurythmics.

   b. "I Will Survive" by Gloria Gaynor.

   c. "Margaritaville" by Jimmy Buffett.

8. If you received a windfall of $100,000, what would you do with it?

   a. Save a third, spend a third on something really special, and give a third to the charity of your choice.

b. Pay off major bills! Then take a trip with the rest.

c. Keep doing what you are doing today, only more of it.

9. Which best describes your handling of monthly bills and expenses?

a. You write checks. What happens after that remains to be seen.

b. You balance the checkbook monthly or your partner/spouse does it.

c. You have a budget and make sure your spending is completely aligned with it.

10. How much of your income do you typically set aside for savings?

a. You can't save anything. You need all your income to live on . . . and then some!

b. You save about 10 percent or more of your income.

c. You save intermittently, when you get a bonus or a tax refund.

Scoring:

For each question, match your answer to the proper score.

1. a, 1; b, 0; c, 2   6.   a, 0; b, 1; c, 2
2. a, 1; b, 0; c, 2   7.   a, 2; b, 1; c, 0
3. a, 0; b, 1; c, 2   8.   a, 1; b, 0; c, 2
4. a, 0; b, 1; c, 2   9.   a, 0; b, 1; c, 2
5. a, 0; b, 2; c, 1   10. a, 0; b, 2; c, 1

Add up your score and check the key below.

0 to 6: Fit to Survive. You're living paycheck to paycheck. You may even be one of the 40 percent of Americans who are living on 110 percent of their income! That also means

---

Bottom-Line Results from Becoming Financially Fit to Live to Enjoy

■ You'll trim your waist as you reduce your debt.

■ You'll maintain good health while you avoid high credit card debt.

■ You'll avoid distress-induced Health Destruction—stress overeating, drinking, social withdrawal, depression, sedentary behavior—brought on by financial challenges.

■ You'll be able to pay for a long and joyful life.

you're living Body Dollar paycheck to Body Dollar paycheck. It's time for the big wake-up call. If you're going to all the trouble to eat better and get exercise, then what's the point if you don't have enough money to buy the gym shoes and healthy foods, as well as the medical insurance to live long and well? Do you live in one of the 44 percent of US households today that does not have enough life insurance to cover the financial loss of a breadwinner? It's time to start saving as many Bank Dollar reserves as your Body Dollar reserves. Health and Wealth management are intertwined for your whole life. Change now and you won't become one of the 65 percent of people who postpone their retirement because they do not have enough money saved.

7 to 13: Fit to Enjoy. You got the Health and Wealth management memo, read it, and are smart enough to have banked enough currency to live healthfully, have fun, and have enough reserves and insurance to weather life's tough challenges. Well done! You are hitting the basic essentials to finance a healthy and enjoyable life journey, and then some. Now, step up to the plate and try to challenge yourself even further. How about that private foundation you could establish to help the needy, or giving to a college or a special group close to your heart?

14 to 20: Fit to Challenge. You're not satisfied just hitting the mark for financial security. All along you've been planning to do something special, over the top with your wealth. You've kept yourself on a financial diet, strategically planning to use your wealth to allow your loved ones and special groups to benefit from your smart saving. You have significant reserves. You are someone who is grateful and a giver via private charities and/or your own foundation. You are willing and can take risks in your career—perhaps you've started your own company—and in your investments. The bottom line is you get it with the life-sustaining connection between Health and Wealth management, and you live it.

CHAPTER 11

The Food Court's Not the Only Place to Binge at the Mall

*"When women are depressed, they eat or go shopping.
Men invade another country."*
—ELAYNE BOOSLER

When we talked about nutrition and exercise, we looked at body composition. You learned that in order to optimize your body comp, you needed to know how much body fat you were carrying around, and then to get down to the business of trimming fat and building muscle to achieve the healthiest body. Well, the same goes for your wallet. Trimming debt is like trimming fat; building wealth is like building muscle. To become Financially Fit to Live, you'll work on creating Bank Dollar reserves, working toward an optimal "financial body composition."

As you read through this chapter, you'll learn that people who are Fit to Live treat Body Dollars and Bank Dollars the same way. When you incorporate the Fit to Live plan into your financial life, you'll also be:

1. *Counting* (calories; currency), *staying accountable* (checking body fat and weight on a scale; reading and tracking your bank statements), and occasionally *spending* (when you succumb to Toxic Stress and waste Body Dollars; when you indulge in excessive retail therapy)
2. *Accruing reserves* (increased physical fitness to use when you must run to save your life; extra cash to weather a divorce, job change, or expensive medical therapies)
3. *Long-term planning* (committing to walk or run a 5-K; creating a will and discussing your financial plan with key family members)
4. *Investing* (walking burns calories, and you build Body Dollar reserves; writing a check for the new pair of walking sneakers allows you to stay active)

Now it's time to learn how we got to an equally troubling place with our finances as we did with our health. In this chapter, you'll learn why it's so easy to run into financial problems—and what you can do to become and stay Financially Fit to Live.

⇨ Our Toxic Lifestyle ⇦
Ballooning Credit Lines to Match Our Waistlines

"I'm living so far beyond my means that we
may almost be said to be living apart."
—E. E. CUMMINGS

Credit has been around since the ancient Egyptians and Babylonians 3,000 years ago. But for most of civilization, we lived within our means, even if that meant hand to mouth—or we went to debtors' prison! The modern credit card was born in 1950, when an embarrassed businessman didn't have the cash to pay for his dinner. Voilà! The Diner's Club card. An explosion of cards followed.

Despite the availability of credit, however, savings exceeded spending for most of our history. Until the 1990s, Americans saved anywhere from 7.5 percent to 14.5 percent of their income, averaging 8 percent. All of a sudden, our savings rate began to drop. Between 2001 and 2004, the US rate was about 1 percent, and in 2005, it went to minus 0.5 per-

> ## "Money often costs too much."
> —*Ralph Waldo Emerson*

cent, the lowest level in history, except for during the 2 worst years of the Depression. What that means is that we are now spending $1.50 for every $1 we make. Uh oh.

To do this, of course, our credit card balances have climbed sky-high. Kind of like our waistlines, our blood pressure, and our glucose levels. The average credit card debt is now over $8,000 per household. Over 50 percent of us handle large or unexpected expenses by using a credit card. Both our credit card debt and our mortgage debt take up higher percentages of our income than ever before, and the number of people who have late payments of over 60 days has ballooned along with our Toxic Belly Fat.

Isn't it interesting that right now, just when we are supposed to live the longest life spans in the history of American culture, we are ending up with the least amount of Bank Dollars to pay for all these extra years?

And what happens once we get that rude awakening when our money runs out? Why stress, of course!

What about you? How's your Financial Fitness? Do you spend less than you make? Do you pay off those credit cards every month? Do you have money in a savings account for a rainy day, like a job layoff? If you're like most folks, the answer to these questions is no. And chances are that the resulting distress is leading you down that thorny road to a ton of dangerous Toxic Belly Fat.

The number one reason we are financially unfit, say experts, is that people are living beyond their means. We're also not asking ourselves the right questions when we purchase

Fascinating FAToid

What Are You Doing at the Office?

One in four American workers at all income levels report serious or overwhelming stress over their finances and struggle to pay their bills. As many as 80 percent admit that at the office, rather than working, they spend a great deal of time worrying about their money woes and dealing with personal financial matters—calling debt collectors, balancing their checkbook, etc. Three million people a year contact a nonprofit credit counseling service looking for help. **Bottom line:** Financial worries can lead to stress-eating.

Fascinating FAToid

The Fat/Money Connection Is Real

If you are obese and female, it's almost twice as likely that you've never had a job, compared with someone of normal weight. **Bottom line:** It's not fair, but whether you stress-eat because you can't find a job, or can't get a job because you're obese from your stress-eating, it's leading to a vicious cycle of distress and health-destruction.

20-foot TV screens, or fridges big enough to feed a small nation. What do these purchases do to our ability to become Fit to Live? Do they foster interest in getting up and moving, or sitting on our rear ends stuffing face? Are we planning how to put aside some Bank Dollars to pay for yoga lessons or cooking classes? When most people develop a budget—if they do one at all—the costs of healthy living are often not taken into consideration. And they're the first thing to go when finances get tight.

Always consider Body Dollars when you're about to spend Bank Dollars, and vice versa. From cars to stoves, it works. If you do, you'll be less likely to pack on the pounds over your lifetime.

Because we don't yet think this way, we keep buying stuff we can't pay for. Just like fast-food restaurants everywhere tempt us to eat mountains of food that aren't good for us, so do miles of mega-malls everywhere tempt us to overspend. So does the fact that everyone takes credit cards, even the IRS. One in 20 of us, both male and female, are shopaholics. Some folks do it to distract themselves from difficult feelings, others do it to show off, still others to gain love. Finally, there are the compulsive hunters, who buy things they don't need because "I got a good deal." Experts say that just like overeating, shopping addiction is growing, due to the availability of credit cards at younger ages, the 24/7 of e-commerce, and TV shopping channels. It's not unusual for compulsive shoppers to have $25,000 in credit card debt, and most have some other psychological problem, usually depression. Like many of us are with our bodies, we are dissociated from our financial reality.

In a national Harris poll of women, most noted that if they had an extra 2 hours,

> "I don't have a bank account because I don't know my mother's maiden name."
> —*Paula Poundstone*

TOP REASONS FOR PACKIN' ON FINANCIAL STRESS POUNDS

1. Falling income without cutting expenses

2. Divorce

3. Bad money management

4. Gambling

5. Medical expenses

6. No reserves for unexpected expenses

7. Inability to talk about money to family members

8. Counting on a windfall

9. Lack of understanding of how money works

If you're in debt, take a look at this list and figure out which ones apply to you. Then make a plan to cut the Financial Debt Fat. If you need help, try the nonprofit Consumer Credit Counseling Service. Go to www.cccsintl.org.

they'd do something wonderful for themselves. What would they do? Why eat and shop, of course! Shopping ranks in the top five recreational activities of the female gender. Hey, there's nothing wrong with the occasional bit of retail therapy, just like the occasional sweet treat. Just put some thought into it, and keep it a treat. Always consider Body Dollars along with Bank Dollars.

One reason experts give for our high credit card debt is that we have high expectations for the future, and figure that we can pay it off later. I don't think so. Living on tomorrow's (imagined) income is never a good idea. That's the kind of thinking that also has us stressed out of our minds, eating poorly, and not exercising now because *someday*, we'll take care of ourselves. Let's get control of those excess pounds and excess debt. What are you waiting for? If not now, *when*?

Why should we cut our Financial Fat? Two reasons—first, if we don't trim our spending habits like our eating habits, we can easily get in way over our heads, gaining so much Toxic Debt that we have no choice but to declare bankruptcy. Think it can't happen? Over

1.5 million families have to do it each year. Researchers talk about bankruptcy boomeranging, which means that many people do it more than once. The new bankruptcy

> "Never spend your money before you have it."
> —*Thomas Jefferson*

laws are complicated, but in general, they require you to give all your money after allowable expenses (determined by the IRS, not you, so your real expenses could be more) to a court trustee, who pays it to your creditors. Plus, there are all kinds of debts, like child support, that it doesn't wipe out. It also ruins your credit for years. It's not a good thing unless you have no other options. If you want help thinking through the issue, go to www.nolo.com.

The other reason we need to cut the Financial Fat is because debt has such a negative effect on the other elements of the Fit to Live lifestyle. Feeling stressed over money creates an inability to concentrate and more fights with family and friends and health destruction.

DO YOU NEED TO REIN IN AN URGE TO SPLURGE?

1. Are you making only minimum payments on your credit cards?
2. When your credit card bill comes, are you surprised to see how much you've spent?
3. Do you have little or no savings?
4. Do you hide purchases or credit card statements from your spouse or lie about what you've bought and spent?
5. Do you buy things on impulse—coming home with stuff you weren't intending to buy?
6. Are your closets and cupboards bulging with stuff you have never used?

If you answer yes to more than one of these questions, you need a program to help you cut the Financial Fat. See my recommendations at the end of the chapter. You might also have a psychological issue you need to address—maybe shopping addiction, depression, or even bipolar disorder. Be sure to seek help if you need it: Follow the links to www.debtorsanonymous.org.

Couples fight over money more than anything else, whether they divorce or stay together. What's the conflict about? Debt and lack of savings causes much more conflict than over-spending, not having enough income, or investing.

My own patients report that the number one stressor in their relationships and cause for divorce is money. And if you get divorced, that's a big-time budget strain. Financial stress is also linked to health woes like depression, anxiety, and insomnia, as well as all the other stress-related illnesses you learned about in Chapter 4—heart problems, weakened immune systems, and premature aging. Forty to 50 percent of people say their health is negatively affected due to financial stress. There's even research that when you respond to money stress with denial and avoidance, you're more likely to get gum disease! Talk about the mind-body connection in action.

Blowing off self-care and health-destruction are such common responses to financial woes that it would be irresponsible of me as a physician not to include money as a key to being Fit to Live. Is money stress a problem for you? How do you respond? Overeating, drinking, smoking, going to the Dark Place, stopping your workouts? Whatever your Bot-

Voice of Success: "It's about So Much More Than Losing Weight."

Helen Stefan owns her own company and had her second child 14 months ago

"When my company was first taking off, I was having lunches every day with clients and gained a lot of weight. After having two children, I realized I had to deal with it. One thing I've learned is that there's such a relationship between Health and Wealth management. Just like balancing your checkbook, you have to balance food and exercise. Just like I want high-quality customers and employees to give me good money results, I want high-quality food and exercise to get good health results. It's really made a difference being able to afford high-quality food and the help of a trainer and nutritionist. I now work out 1 hour a day. That's non-negotiable. I'm in size 8s, down from 14s. But what's truly amazing is my energy level. I have energy for my kids, my company, my husband, myself. Becoming Fit to Live is about so much more than losing weight."

Fascinating FATroid

Why Cut Credit Card Fat?

In England, the majority of people named money as the number one factor in their quality of life, with health second, and crime a distant third. A US survey found that the majority of women list money as their primary worry (30 percent), ahead of weight (20 percent), job (12 percent), and health (11 percent). What's keeping them awake at night? Debt. **Bottom line:** Manage your money well, and you'll be able to manage your stress, sleep, and waistline!

tom Feeding behaviors happen to be, your lack of dollars in the bank will end up creating a huge debt in Body Dollars too.

I'm not Suze Orman. I'm a doctor helping you make the Bank Dollar/Body Dollar connection. I'm not going to give you the detailed advice you'd get from a financial planner. But with the help of my friends at Prudential Financial, with whom I've done a lecture series on Health and Wealth management for women, called Stepping Out, I'm offering the five basic principles of Financial Fitness as well as my Fit to Live Essentials to make sure you are as Fit in Money as you are becoming in Mind, Mouth, and Muscle.

⇒Fit to Live⇐
Living within Our Means

"If money be not thy servant, it will be thy master."
—FRANCIS BACON

I know from years of experience that there's a strong relationship between Health and Wealth management. When I say wealth, I don't expect you to be a multimillionaire. I just mean whatever wealth you have, even if it's $30,000 a year, make sure you're managing it in such a way that it helps you be Fit to Live. The better you are at managing your money, the better you'll be at managing your health. And vice versa. That's because it takes similar planning and tracking. A Prudential survey confirms my belief—about half of women say that it is equally difficult to maintain or improve their health and wealth.

> "The art of living easily as to money is to pitch your scale of living one degree below your means."
>
> —*Sir Henry Taylor*

Folks who are Fit to Live understand this relationship and have their financial houses in order to save their own lives if need be. They strive to pay off their credit cards monthly, have the Mental Fitness to say no to purchases they can't afford, and have savings for emergencies and for retirement (more on the last in the next chapter).

Research shows that Money Fitness leads to success in healthy living. The more money you make, for instance, the more active you are likely to be. Even taking out access to health care, the more money you make, the healthier you are. And the more money you have, the less likely you are to be obese. With one exception: African American men's obesity rate actually rises as their income does. (So guys, be careful. Don't let your waistline grow with your bank account. Get the Mind, Mouth, and Muscle going too.)

Want more proof of the Mind-Mouth-Muscle-Money connection? Forty-three percent of folks who join a debt management program report their health improved shortly after. So, are you ready to take yourself on and bank those Bank Dollars as well as Body Dollars? With Mouth and Muscle, it's all about eating less and moving more, right? In Money, it's all about spending less and saving more.

THE FIVE FIT TO LIVE SPEND LESS, SAVE MORE PRINCIPLES

1. Know the Meaning of Your Money

What really matters to you when it comes to money? Go back to the Power Why you created in Chapter 2. The more you know what motivates you, the more you can line up your money priorities to match. For instance, if your mission is to be the best parent possible, use that to say no to overspending so you won't be a financial burden on your kids. Or perhaps your mission is to save money for their college education. Or to make a difference in the world. Can you do that if you are stressed out all the time about money? Your Power Why for money helps you focus on your values.

I first began to understand the importance of values in relation to money while filming my Discovery Health TV show, "The National Body Challenge." I'd ask people to walk, and they'd say "sneakers are expensive." Then I'd look around the house and see lots of junk food, a TV in every room (including a wide screen), every electronic gadget known to mankind, and mountains of CDs. It's funny how there's money for these big-ticket items and yet no money to join a gym, buy the appropriate food, go to that yoga class, or attend Weight Watchers. Put your money where your true values are. Your Power Why can help.

Keeping your mission front and center also helps distinguish between wants and needs, which is key to being Fit to Live, whether you're tempted by a giant hot pastrami sandwich or those pair of Manolo Blahniks that are calling your name. You may *want* them, but do you really *need* that food or a pair of shoes right now? If you really do have a need, how can you fill it in a way that causes the least health- and self-destruction in Body and Bank Dollars? Debt counselors say that people spend money unconsciously, to escape problems. Sounds like the mindless eating we do, right? When our priorities are front and center, we're more mindful of our choices.

2. Own Your Financial Fitness

Have you offloaded the financial tasks to your spouse? It's okay if one person takes on the primary task of balancing the checkbook or paying the bills. But that doesn't mean you blow it off entirely.

I can't tell you the number of female patients of mine who left the money up to their husbands and then had rude awakenings after their husbands' deaths. Second mortgages taken out without their knowing it, secret boat purchases, borrowing against home equity lines of credit or stock options, and in one case, a purchase of another home without the wife's awareness. Some women are so unaware that they don't even know if he had a life insurance policy or where the financial documents are! This terrible financial stress usually leads to health-destruction and the buildup of that Toxic Belly Fat, which will eventually lead to the stress of new medical conditions.

Don't leave your financial well-being in someone else's hands, even a spouse. You need to have full disclosure to be Financially Fit to Live. Financial infidelity is all too real. Three-quarters of men and 67 percent of women come into marriage with debt. Over half of those folks owe more than $5,000, mostly from car and student loans, as well as credit cards. One partner might not want to deliver that bad news at the beginning of their lives together. Or perhaps one spouse is a com-

> "Proportion your expenses to what you have, not what you expect."
> —*English proverb*

pulsive shopper and doesn't want the other to know how large the credit card balances are. Or he has a secret account in order to avoid a large settlement in the case of a breakup.

Perhaps there is no bad intention at all. One patient of mine had a husband who was just plain disorganized. He never created a budget, so he didn't realize that the new jobs they had both taken had serious pay cuts, which meant they were going in the hole to the tune of $500 per month, depleting their emergency savings. She didn't know how much trouble they were in until a year later, when their cable service was cut off and their savings account was empty. Her response to the resulting financial distress packed on 30 pounds around her waist.

Avoid monetary shock as well as health-destruction by keeping on top of your financial reality. Know where all your accounts are and what's in 'em. Don't just "trust." Own it.

3. Arm Yourself with Information

Just because you need to take responsibility for your Financial Fitness doesn't mean you have to figure it all out on your own. Just like you might need support in Mind, Mouth, or Muscle, you may need help in this important area. One in four Americans lacks confidence in their capacity to manage their finances. Women are more involved in financial decision-making than they were 5 years ago, but 62 percent are still uncertain whether they are on the right path to meet their financial goals. They feel they lack the knowledge, the confidence, and the time to make the right choices. Only one in five feels prepared to make Financially Fit decisions.

Of course, we lack confidence. Most of us have not been taught even the basics of personal finance. It is complicated. But you read *Prevention* and *Men's Health*, or *Health* and *Fitness* magazines to be up on the latest Mouth and Muscle Fitness, don't you? Well, no difference here. Get the info that will help you be Financially Fit. Attend a free course on basic finances. Ask a friend for a referral to a financial advisor. Read the *New York Times* personal finance section. Or *Money* magazine. Or go online to SmartMoney.com or Bankrate.com for all kinds of free, objective information. The more you know, the better decisions you'll make.

4. Face the Music about Your Unfitness

How can you get Fit to Live if you don't admit how unfit you are? Six out of 10 women say they put as much energy into their wealth as their health. Given how unfit we are, that's not good news. One-quarter of men and women don't even look at their credit card statements when they come in to see where the money is being spent. Just like the folks who can't tell you their blood pressure or cholesterol. Whether it's Bank Dollars or Body Dollars, you need to stay informed and accountable.

Do you know what your monthly expenses are? Do you have any idea how much credit card debt you have? If you aren't paying the balance each month, have you calculated how long it will take to pay off and how much you need to put toward it each month? Do you know your credit score, which is a measure of whether you pay your bills on time, and influences not only whether you will get a loan for a car or home, but also what interest rate you'll be charged and sometimes even whether you'll get a job?

Do you know how much you have in savings? Over 40 percent of women have less than $500 in the bank. Information is key to Financial Fitness, as is taking action on the information once you get the facts. Just like a business needs a profit/loss statement, you need to know your income versus your expenses, plus the total you owe. To do this, you need a strong mind, one that is willing to take the necessary actions to get Financially Fit. You may have to get a second job, sell excess stuff on e-Bay, or get a roommate. But you can't A^2 it until you first tell yourself your True Truth and face your current financial reality. It's like finally measuring your waist and facing that number. Take yourself on, acknowledge the pain, and face the music. Then you can save your life—Mentally, Physically, and now Financially.

5. Wake Up and Realize What Money Really Buys

There's only one thing money buys you—options. It does not buy you happiness. This is so true for weight as well. Dropping weight does not guarantee you a terrific life. But like money, it gives you more options—more attractive clothes to wear, a better chance for the job you wanted, and a decreased risk of disease and disability.

Fascinating FAToid

Know Your Body Fat *and* Your Interest Rate

Seven in 10 of us have at least one credit card. But 34 percent of us who do have no idea what the interest rate is on the card we use most often. If you pay off your balance every month, then it's not an issue. But if not, you really should know. There's great variation, and depending on your balance, you could be paying significant dollars. **Bottom line:** Avoid being mindless about the critical factors that determine your ability to become Financially Fit to Live.

"Why is there so much month left at the end of the money?"

—*Anonymous*

In both cases, however, the more money you make and the better physical shape you're in will definitely increase your satisfaction with life—up to a point. Researchers found that 56 percent of people who make more than $75,000 a year say they are "very satisfied" with their life. Only 24 percent of people who make $25,000 or less a year say they are.

But here's the catch. Once basic needs are met, then more money didn't make anyone any more satisfied. Forty-two percent of people who made $50,000 to $89,000 a year feel "very happy." Only 43 percent of people who made $90,000 or more a year felt the same.

Turns out there's been no change in the overall level of happiness from the year 1957, when the average after-tax income was $10,171, to 1980, when the income was $17,931, or 2004, when the income was $27,237. In each year, the level of happiness was 34 percent. We make more money, then adapt to that level of living and wish for more.

You need to ask yourself what really makes you truly happy. Surveys have found that health and home win over accumulating more "stuff." Here's the rundown:

84 percent: good health

60 percent: owning your home

48 percent: children

46 percent: a good job

36 percent: leisure time

22 percent: gardening

19 percent: some luxury or a nice second car

19 percent: the latest gadgets

Go back to your Power Why. If you're telling yourself that friends and family are the main focus of your life, then why are you desperately seeking happiness from that next raise or scoring that hot new car?

⇨Fit to Live Essentials⇦

Using your score from the "Are You Financially Fit to Live?" test, you'll continue to build your individual program with the tips below. As in previous chapters, you'll begin according to your current level.

TO SURVIVE:

If you received a score of 0 to 6 on the test, focus your energy here first. Once you've mastered these, feel free to move up to the tips in "To Enjoy."

1. Get Going with Great Goals

People who set goals have been found to be more satisfied and wealthier 20 years later than those who didn't. Use your Power Why to help you decide what matters most to you, then make a plan to achieve that. Just as you did with your health priorities earlier in the book, it's time to get clear about your financial expectations.

Sit down with your spouse, or do this with a friend if you live alone. Ask the other person, "What's important about money to you?" Imagine they say something like, "It gives me security." Then ask, "What's important about security to you?" No matter what they say, ask them what's important about that to them until they get to their bottom-line values. Then switch and have them do it for you. The trick when you are the asker is to stay completely quiet except for asking the question. Once you have what really matters to you, make a budget based on your priorities. A patient of mine did this and discovered what was important to her was exploring other cultures. That made it easier for her to say no to mall temptations and sock away money in a travel fund.

2. Track Your Currency Just Like Your Calories

Winging it with finances is as dangerous to your health as winging eating and exercise. Just like you're now tracking what you're eating and how much you're moving, you've got to track your money. And that means creating a budget and then recording expenses on a regular basis. If you've never made a budget before in your life, and you don't know how, go to the Consumer Credit Counseling Service at www.cccsatl.org and click on "CCCS calculators" to access their budget calculator. This tool not only helps you figure out what you're spending, but also gives recommendations of how much you should be spending in each category.

Tracking your expenses allows you to really understand where your money is going so you can make different choices in alignment with being Fit to Live. You may be surprised to discover how much you're spending on fast food or lattes. If you smoke, how much is that little habit costing? Want to join a gym? How much do you need to set aside for the monthly membership fee? You can't trim your Toxic Belly Fat if you don't make sound money decisions for your health.

Fascinating FAToid

Trouble Tightening Your Money Belt?

Try this practice for cutting impulse purchases: Carry a piece of paper in your wallet. Every time you see something you want, write it down on the paper and tell yourself that if you still want it in a week, you can buy it. Here's the trick—you can have only four items on your list at any one time. If you see something else you want, you've got to cross something off your list. **Bottom line:** What you may discover is that just like with the impulse to gobble an entire chocolate cake, the urge to buy those jeans is short lived.

3. Cut Credit Card Fat

Do you have balances you can't pay? Do you use one card to pay off another? Did you take out a home equity loan to pay off credit cards only to find your balances are sky-high again? You can easily be paying up to 25 percent interest on those cards.

Cutting credit card fat is crucial for overall Financial Fitness. Just like trimming body fat consists of both eating right and moving more, there are two parts to trimming credit card fat: paying off the balances you now have and not accumulating more.

Add up the total of what you owe in credit card debt. Having a wake-up call yet? Time to A². Look at your budget and see how much you can afford to put toward your debt each month. Figure out how long you will need to keep at it till you get to zero. If you have more than one card, start with the one with the highest rate. Tackle it just like body weight, be patient and steady. Be sure to get the payments in on time; otherwise you get hit with late fees and penalty rates that are as high as 30 percent on your total. That's how a small amount can get out of control fast. Also, switch to cards with the lowest interest—www.cardweb.com has the facts. Get help from a credit counseling service if it seems too overwhelming. A good free one is Consumer Credit Counseling Services: www.cccsintl.org.

To stop adding to the damage, cut up all but one credit card, and call the companies to cancel your account. Stash your remaining card in the freezer, so you'll have to thaw it to use it! Then, go cash only—it's one of the very best ways to rein in spending. Use a debit card or an old-fashioned check for those times you find yourself without cash in your pocket.

4. Quit Wearing Your Nest Egg, and Start Saving Your Life

Life happens. Like me, you might break an ankle. If you're in good shape beforehand, you're able to maintain your body comp. But if you've been asleep at the meal, the problem is much worse. The same is true for finances. Are you in good enough financial shape to weather a crisis? When things happen—and they will—you'll have to pay in Body Dollars and Bank Dollars. That's why everyone should have a reserve.

The peace of mind you get from not living from paycheck to paycheck is profound. More than 70 percent of folks say they worried about their finances in the past year, usually because of unexpected expenses like car repairs or a leaky roof. We're financing such things with our credit cards because we have no emergency savings. Plus, with all the constant layoffs going on, job security isn't what it used to be. Financial planners say it's smart to have enough money for months of job-hunting.

That means you've got to take the money you've been spending and start putting it into a savings or money market account. I've seen recommendations everywhere from $1,000 for emergencies such as flying to visit a sick parent to 4 to 6 months of salary. My thought? Whatever amount will help you stay out of Bottom Feeding. Just like you build a reserve of Body Dollars one good choice at a time, so you can build a reserve of Bank Dollars.

Here's a great way. Have a set amount deducted from your paycheck and deposited into a savings account. What you don't see, you don't miss. Even if it's only $50 or $100, it can really add up over time. If you wait until the money lands in your checking account, it's too easy to spend it—often on unnecessary treats that add to your waistline. Consider a high interest checking account that has no fees and no minimums, like ING Direct or the

Fascinating FAToid

Is Fear of Being a Bag Lady Showing Up on Your Waistline?

Almost half of us women have fears of becoming financially destitute, even those in the highest income brackets. That's why two-thirds say the best thing about having money is feeling secure. Men are much less fearful. That may be why women are twice as likely as men to have a secret stash of money. **Bottom line:** When women feel more financially secure, they're less likely to stress-eat.

online bank HSBC. The interest rates are higher than some brick-and-mortar banks, and you can take your money out at any time with no penalty. When you hit the emergency savings goal you're going for, it's time to consider investing. We'll tackle that in the next chapter.

5. Box Your Bank Dollar Documents

Becoming Financially Fit to Live also means you have all the records you need and you know where they are. And you let other people know too, in case something happens to you. Fill out the Document Locator form in Appendix 4 or download it from my Web site, www.drpeeke.com. (Be sure to keep the paper in a secure place, like a safe deposit box—it gives someone ready access to your very important info—and give a copy to a trusted friend.)

To fill out the form, you'll have to find all the pertinent papers and decide where to put them, which may take time. But it's a one-time deal. If you've already got your papers organized, it will take only a few minutes to write down where they are. If you are married, it's a great thing to do together so that you'll both know where everything is.

TO ENJOY:

If you scored a 7 to 13 on the test, just take a quick look at the "To Survive" suggestions. If you feel you have them covered, you can start here.

1. Create the Piggy Bank of Joy

Recycle a pretty jar for your piggy bank of joy. Fill it with your extra change. Search your car, your couches, under the bed, and in old purses for all that spare change. Have the kids look. Experts say we have around $100 lying around in coins. Next, write down things that you could do with that money that really give you joy—a trip to visit friends, a body sculpting class, a new iPod to keep you company when you walk, a pet. Start saving a few dollars a week toward the goal of "joying" yourself. Whenever you have a choice to buy something, ask yourself, Do I really need that or should this be another deposit in the "piggy bank of joy?"

2. Make the Health-Wealth Connection a Win/Win

Before you make any purchase, ask yourself, How will this affect my health and wellness? Will this lead to Toxic Belly Fat? Buying a book of puzzles or Sudoku? That wealth expenditure just increased your mental acuity and decreased your chances for memory loss and dementia. Purchasing a home with a garden and extra room for your exercise equipment? It's the best kind of return on investment. Two-for-one at Cinnabon? Not so much.

3. Give Bank Dollars Straight from Your Heart

What really matters to you? Ending hunger? Taking care of abandoned animals? Experience the pleasure of giving on a regular basis to something important to you. A wonderful way to show your joy is to share it with others who need your financial help.

TO CHALLENGE

If you scored a 14 to 20 on the test, just take a quick look at the "To Survive" and "To Enjoy" tips. If you feel you have them covered, you can start here.

1. Pay Down Your Mortgage

Got extra cash every month? After you have a solid savings plan in place (see Chapter 12), consider putting it toward the principle on your mortgage. You will be surprised at how that might cut down on its remaining years. By putting in $500 extra a month, one patient of mine paid off a 30-year mortgage in 22 years. Any amount on a regular basis helps.

2. Start a 529 College Fund for Your Child or Grandchild

These are state-sponsored college savings plans. If your child doesn't go to college, another family member (including you) can use it for higher education. Get details at www.savingforcollege.com.

3. Become a Philanthropist

Once you're at the Fit to Live to Challenge level, you're in the special position of giving back through the establishment of your own foundation. Sit down with your financial planner or accountant and discuss your goals. Whether you want to give to your alma mater or to a special interest group, giving back is a wonderful way to generate happiness, joy, and a feeling of achievement.

CHAPTER 12

Don't Retire—
Refire and Rejoice!

"I have enough money to last me the rest of my life,
unless I buy something."
—JACKIE MASON

Today, the word *retirement* is actually outdated. This term applied to a time when the life span was shorter. We now live longer and are able to continue to be creative and productive long after the traditional retirement age. My good friend Kenneth Cooper, MD, founder of the Cooper Aerobics Institute, who is in his mid-seventies and still at the helm of his empire, noted that he does not believe in the word *retire*. He likes "refire." Ken believes this is a time in life to get excited, reinvent yourself, and keep the energy of life flowing in you. Amen, Ken!

"Refirement." I like the sound of that. You say the word and immediately think of the endless opportunities to fire it up and transition from one level of living to another. The gold medal winners in longevity, the centenarians, are famous for living lives that are intellectually and physically active. They transition from decade to decade, weathering life's storms, and keep stoking that fire of life.

Like those centenarians, we want to stay Alert and Vertical for as long as we can. We cannot be only Mentally, Nutritionally, and Physically Fit to Live to get the most out of our day-to-day lives, but we also need to have the Body Dollars and Bank Dollars to weather the physical and financial challenges of aging and enjoy our lives to the fullest.

Do you have enough money to fund your "refirement"? Laying down a strong financial foundation will enable you to live a healthy lifestyle, knowing that the tab can be paid.

⇒Our Toxic Lifestyle⇐
The Future Isn't So Rosy

"I don't like money, but it quiets my nerves."
—JOE LOUIS

For most of human history, saving for the traditional retirement made no sense, even if you could afford to—it wasn't likely that you would live long enough to need a stockpile. You worked until you died, usually quite young. If you were one of the lucky few who made it into old age, your retirement plan could be summed up in one word: family. Ditto for your disability plan and your life insurance plan.

How did parents get their kids to take care of them? Promising them the farm, literally! But as opportunities for work grew in cities, kids started bailing. So, beginning in the 19th century, the military started providing pensions, and companies soon followed. Then, in 1935, when over 50 percent of senior citizens were living in poverty, the government instituted Social Security to provide retirement and disability income and, in 1965, created the Medicare system, to provide health insurance to the elderly and disabled.

Want to know what a big change these things made? In 1840, 76.6 percent of men over 65 worked. In 2000, that number was only 17.5 percent. Retirement has now become a significant phase of life for the majority of people. And Social Security and pensions are now the main source of retirement income of the elderly population.

"Money is like a sixth sense without which you cannot make a complete use of the other five."
—W. Somerset Maugham

If you're reading this and assuming this is the scenario going into the future, you're in for a rude awakening. Pensions are becoming a rarity, and Social Security funds may run out. How did that happen?

First, people started living longer. When Social Security was instituted, the average life expectancy was 61.1 years. Most people didn't live long enough to even qualify! Second, there are more people than anticipated who will need Social Security. The famous Baby Boom of the '50s and '60s resulted in a huge bulge of people who've been working for decades, paying into the system. Starting in 2006, we began to retire, and there will not be enough money to pay us all what we're owed. The estimate from the Social Security Administration is that by 2041, it will only have 74 percent of what it needs to pay eligible folks. Desperate for a remedy, some folks intended to take investments more seriously. But did they? In 2004, 53 percent of those polled planned to invest more money that year, but by 2006, only 11 percent had.

To make matters worse, Medicare projects it will run out of money by 2018—just more than a decade away, folks—for similar reasons. Finally, many corporations that had been offering guaranteed pensions are stopping, some due to bankruptcy and others because they see it as a cost they can't afford. Instead, a lot of companies are offering 401ks. In 1978, only 17 percent of workers had such a plan; today, 56 percent do.

As a result of these unfortunate facts, 40 percent of Americans are really stressed out about their retirement years. These folks think it is very unlikely they will receive their full Social Security benefits. Are you feeling stressed as well? It's time to get armed and dangerous with the right information and a plan to get Financially Fit to Live.

First, you have to know what you need to know. My friend Maria Umbach of Prudential Financial puts it this way: Women obsess about their credit scores like they do about their weight. Yet in both cases, we're focusing on the wrong things. As you've learned, whether you're male or female, your overall weight says nothing about your body composition—whether you have Toxic Belly Fat, strong bones and muscles, optimal physical performance—or whether you have any long-term reserve of Body Dollars to fend off crises. Your credit score says you pay your bills on time—period. It says nothing about whether you're paying those bills by living paycheck to paycheck or whether you have any Bank Dollar reserves to pay for a healthy lifestyle in the future. It's time to A^2 and get focused on those "refirement" reserves.

FOUR MINDSETS TO BECOME FIT FOR REFIREMENT

1. Working Longer Makes Good Cents

Men retire on average at 63 and women at 62. That's *before* full Social Security benefits kick in. Even if you have no retirement savings, say experts, you have to work only 3½ years longer to dodge a big drop-off in your lifestyle. The longer you work, the more money you can save in investments and give them time to grow, and the less time you'll be dipping into retirement savings. To do this, you need to stay mentally and physically fit.

2. In a Divorce, Get Those Retirement Savings

Fight for your half of the 401ks, etc. Women in particular often trade their part of the retirement funds for the family home and then can't afford to live in it. Your life may be pinched later if you make this choice.

3. Pay Yourself before Your Kids

Parents (especially the woman) can get so hung up on taking care of the kids that they can forget about their retirement savings. But children can survive indebtedness better than you because they're younger. They can take out loans to go to college, or work while going to school. They don't have to have the $30,000 wedding, the new car at 16, or the $100,000 private college education. But you do need money for old age.

4. Homeownership Is Smart, Even Later in Life

If you rent, housing accounts for 33.6 percent of your income; homeownership uses only 18.3 percent. Plus, rent can go up each year, and you're not building equity. With ownership, you get equity (if you don't keep borrowing on your house) that you can use in old age through a home equity loan or a reverse mortgage (where you get income from your house while you live in it).

Sixty-nine percent of us have put away money for retirement. So far, so good. But, say experts, not enough money. The average amount in men's 401ks is only $40,703, and women's in only $24,720. Women's are so much less because we still make less money than men and often have shorter work histories due to childrearing and other family duties. That's not good news, because we live longer (3 years on average) and spend more money on health care at the end of our lives. We need the Bank Dollar reserve to match our Body Dollar reserve!

People typically don't think about retirement savings until they are in their fifties, and how much money you make has little to do with whether you are focused on this goal or not. Six in 10 of us are behind schedule—hmm, the same percentage of us that are over-weight or obese . . .

The distress of Bank Dollar debt is indeed associated with Toxic Belly Fat. Almost half of us are resigned to struggling during retirement. That's the helplessness, hopelessness, and defeat of Toxic Stress, which leads so many people to health-destructive behaviors just when they should be enjoying the refirement years. Some experts are saying that the situation is so bad that the traditional retirement age may have to increase by as much as 10 years for people to afford to stop working. That means working until you're 75 or beyond.

But you can't count on working as long as you might want. Four in 10 of us may be forced to retire due to a job loss, family crisis, or disease and disability. What's the solution? Why, it's the same template for every one of our Fit to Live elements, from Mind to Macrocosm. The answer lies in our ability to get a grip on reality, know our current status, seek the right information and resources to guide us, make a plan, and A² it.

⇒Fit to Live⇐

"[R]iches have wings . . . they must be set flying to bring in more."
—FRANCIS BACON

People who are Fit to Live certainly increase the possibility of working as long as they want. But working longer is not their only retirement plan. They've figured out what they will need to fund their future and have taken action to create the necessary funds. They also have been honest with themselves and their loved ones about the realities of

> ## Voice of Success: Daily Focus Maintains Health and Wealth
>
> **Louise Grove went from dress size 16 to 12**
>
> "I was a very successful salesperson in the corporate world, but I became overweight and unfit. So a year ago, I decided to start my own consulting business so I could make being Fit to Live a priority. I plan my meetings and travel around working out. I do 3 to 4 miles a day on the elliptical and lift weights twice a week. I just completed my first 5-mile Race for the Cure walk. I'm halfway to my target weight. And guess what? I'm making more money than ever before, so I am better prepared for retirement. When I worked for others, they set the targets, and I had to deal with their stress. Now I set my own goals. I push myself hard but am able to work on the other things that matter to me. I have the daily focus to maintain my health and my wealth. The structure's there."

disability and death and have made appropriate choices there too. If you are like most people and have avoided these actions, armed with my Five Principles and Fit to Live Essentials that I've created with my friends at Prudential Financial, you'll be well on your way to your optimal refirement.

THE FIVE FIT TO LIVE REFIREMENT FITNESS PRINCIPLES

1. Pay Yourself to Live

At some point, we're not going to get a paycheck from our employer, and we will need to pay ourselves to fund the continuation of our healthy lifestyle. That's what refirement Bank Dollars are really about—income replacement. Even if you do get full Social Security benefits, they won't replace your whole income. How much they replace depends on what you earn. If you earn $30,000 to $40,000 a year, it's going to replace around 60 percent. If you earn $150,000, it will be only between 17 and 25 percent. (See "Get a Refirement Goal" on page 234 for info on how to reach this mark.)

> "Certainly, there are things in life that money can't buy, but it's very funny— did you ever try buying them without money?"
>
> —*Ogden Nash*

How much of your income will you need? More than you think. Experts used to say 75 to 85 percent. Now they are saying you need more like 100 percent. How come? Because we're living longer. In addition, because we're having kids later, 60 percent of today's retirees may still be caring for dependent children in addition to spouses and aging parents. Also because the reduced costs of work expenses—like clothes, commuting, etc.—are more than offset by increased medical costs not covered by Medicare. In 2004, a 45-year-old was spending less than 4 percent of her income on health. By age 75, that number climbs to over 14 percent. Remember, because of all the Body Dollars you're banking, you could live as much as 30 years past 65. You need to be able to fund that.

2. It's Never Too Late to Become Financially Fit

What if you're 40 and just getting the big wake-up call reading this? Or you're almost 50 and thinking, I got wiped out in my divorce and am starting all over again. Or you're a guy who just got laid off at age 55?

Don't despair. It's never too late. It's really no different than when people come to me at age 40 or 50 or 60, overweight or obese, loaded with Toxic Belly Fat, with a mountain of Body Dollar debt. No worries. Take a deep breath, calmly and patiently assess the situation, and get a plan in motion. (See the Fit to Live Essentials on page 233 for advice on how to

Fascinating FAToid

Get Your Mind in Gear

The top five reasons people give for not having enough retirement savings? High expenses, career choice, job loss or frequent job changes, wanting a comfortable lifestyle, and lack of financial discipline. **Bottom line:** Just like with Mouth and Muscle, you've got to get your Mind on your side. This is important stuff, folks. Chances are you're eating out several times a week. Pack a lunch instead of eating out, cook instead of buying convenience foods, and invest the savings to fund a lifetime of healthy living. You'll be wealthier—and healthier!

Fascinating FAToid

Close the Knowledge Gap

About 50 percent of workers don't feel knowledgeable about investing, and most lack even the basics of how a 401k works. **Bottom line:** It's okay not to know, but it's not okay to stay stuck in not knowing. You owe it to your waistline to get help from a financial planner or a basic magazine like *Money* to avoid stress-eating.

get started. The good news is that as you get older, the amount of pre-tax contributions you can put into plans such as 401ks increases.)

Just as the truth of your cholesterol levels can spur you into action mentally, physically, and nutritionally, so can the truth of your IRA level get you going financially. Any Body Dollar or Bank Dollar reserves you can sock away right now will be lifesaving.

3. Know How to Save for the Refirement Years

Thankfully, you have a variety of options for funding your refirement. Let's take a quick look at the biggies.

Pension. Unfortunately, not many of us have much to say in this department these days. The lucky few who still have pensions might not want to depend on them too much— many large companies have rescinded on this once-sacred trust. If you have one, count yourself as lucky—but don't count on it paying out.

401ks. A 401k is a retirement savings and investment plan sponsored by your employer and funded by you with pretax money deducted from your paycheck. There are no minimums. You make your investment choices from a list offered by the plan, based on what kind of risk you are comfortable with and how much time you have. Some employers match some or all of what you put in; if you don't take advantage of that, it's like giving away free money. (If you are self-employed, similar plans are available.) Warning: If you take out any money before retirement, you must generally pay a penalty, plus federal and state taxes.

IRAs. An IRA is an individual retirement account that works similarly. How much money you can put in tax-free depends on your age and other factors, including what kind of IRA it is.

Mutual funds. Whatever the plan, most people invest in mutual funds, rather than individual stocks or bonds. Mutual funds give you the ability to invest in a lot of different companies, with someone else—a professional fund administrator—worrying about what to buy and sell when. You share in the upside potential of the stock market, while being diversified. Every mutual fund has a specific investment objective. There are even green mutual funds for the environmentally conscious. Some funds invest in small companies, so there's more risk but more opportunity for reward. Some invest in companies that have been around forever, which has less upside potential, but you have less risk.

Annuities. Another way to get a retirement income stream is to buy an annuity, which is sold by insurance companies. Here's how it works: Imagine you have $100,000. The insurance company does the math based on mortality and other factors, and says if you give them the $100,000 now, they will guarantee you X amount of money per month or per year, no matter how long you live. So it's guaranteed income. Make sure your insurance company is as Fit to Live as you are. Look for a company that has been around a long time, with a trusted brand, and good ratings from outside rating agencies like AM Best, Moody's, or Standard and Poor's. It needs to be around to pay you for the rest of your life.

A WORD ABOUT INVESTING

Investing, in general, is all about risk and reward. We should buy low and sell high, but too many of us buy when we see others buying (high) and sell when others are selling (low). Too many of us think we can have our cake (high returns) and eat it too (no short-term losses). That's like trying to find a magic weight loss pill that allows us to eat whatever and still shed pounds. It doesn't exist. Rather, just like with trimming your Toxic Belly Fat, you need discipline, accountability, and an understanding of cause and effect to achieve your investment goals.

Fortunately, you don't have to figure this out on your own, people! Balancing risk and reward and rebalancing as you age is what professionals help you do. They can also help you think through the issue of fees and expenses, because funds have a variety of ways of charging you, which you must take into account.

4. Insure Your Fit to Live Lifestyle

Insurance is the kind of thing we all know we need but put off thinking about. Here are the basics. There are four kinds of insurance we need to think about when becoming Fit to Live: health, disability, life, and long-term care. Read the basics here and consult an insurance agent for the best plan for you.

Health insurance. Hopefully right now, you have health insurance through your employer. As I said at the beginning of this chapter, what will happen to Medicare is anyone's guess at this point. Many politicians of both parties still continue to talk about universal health care. Given the ever-changing landscape, I'm not going to suggest anything in this department except that you pay close attention to developments in what's happening with this important future expense. Pay attention to how plans address drug coverage. This is most important after age 40.

Disability insurance. This type of insurance exists to give you income if you get an illness or an injury and can't work. This is much more likely to happen than dying when you're young. One insurance company estimates that one-third of us will have some kind of health crisis before the age of 65 that keeps us from working for 90 days or longer. Can you afford to lose 90 days of income? Disability insurance helps guard against this loss. Your employer and/or Social Security may cover part of this, but you still may have a gap that can be filled by individual disability insurance. Otherwise, you can eat into or destroy your retirement nest egg.

Life insurance. Life insurance exists to make up lost income to your family if you die. Many companies offer this as a benefit, and employees can supplement the policy. If you're

Fascinating FAToid

Planning for Hardship

Seventy-one percent of Americans are very or somewhat concerned about needing long-term care in the future, 74 percent have had experience with a family member needing care, and almost as many recognize that long-term care insurance is important to their family's financial security. But only 21 percent have bought the insurance. When asked what they planned to do, responses included: "nothing," "hope and pray," "wait for the government to do something." **Bottom line:** Just like with your health, it's time to take action!

> "I detest life-insurance
> agents. They always argue
> that I shall someday die,
> which is not so."
>
> —*Stephen Leacock*

a stay-at-home spouse, don't fall into the trap of thinking you don't need life insurance. You may be amazed to discover how much your duties are worth. In 2006, it would cost a working husband $134,000 a year if his wife passed away and he had to replace what she did: running the kids to soccer, doing the grocery shopping, managing the household, and so on. That's something, huh? You can find out what it would cost to replace your services at "All You Do" at www.prudential.com.

Long-term care insurance. Long-term care insurance pays for assisted living care, whether that's in a nursing home or having somebody come to your home. It's estimated that more than half of us will need some kind of long-term care, eventually. And we all know which half—women! It's, of course, a generalization, but men tend to go quickly and women linger. Without insurance, unless you are very poor to begin with, you're going to start depleting your savings. If you do have to go into a nursing home, estimates are that you will have to pay as much on average as $61,000 a year out of pocket. No matter how many Body Dollars you bank, as you age, the mathematical probability of picking up some debilitating disease increases precipitously. So you've got to be prepared for it.

One of the main reasons we don't get long-term care insurance is that we're in denial of what shape we're going to be in when we're older. A patient of mine told me about talking with her mother when her father needed to be put in a nursing home. Her mom was terrified he would go through the savings she would need to live on and was stress-eating over this and piling on the Toxic Belly Fat, ramping up her own blood pressure and blood sugars. When my patient asked if they had long-term care insurance, her mother explained, "No, we decided that whoever was sick would be taken care of by the other. But I never expected to be so old when I had to do it."

Here's another myth that gets in our way of buying long-term care insurance: Don't worry, Medicare will pay for everything. Even if it's still in existence as it is today, that's not true. It actually pays only part of the costs. And to qualify for Medicaid, you have to spend down all your assets to about $2,000. People living in poverty will be covered. High-income people who have enough assets don't have to worry. It is middle-income folks who are the ones who most need this particular safety net.

Life, long-term care insurance, and disability are paid in Body Dollars, or lack thereof. Meaning you pay more if you are unfit, or if you're really unfit, you may not

> "Money is a terrible master but an excellent servant."
> —*Phineas Taylor Barnum*

be able to get coverage. Both life and long-term care insurance also get more expensive to buy the older you get. So don't procrastinate on this one—experts advise getting long-term care insurance at around 50.

5. Start on Your Refirement Plan Now

Special message for women: Don't overthink this, just do it. Now. You don't have to think about how you're going to do it and why you haven't done it, and when's the perfect time to bring it up with your husband, and all the articles you have to read before you can start, and the color-coded file folders you need to buy. . . . Remember, women are innately hardwired to ruminate and overplan in an attempt to do it perfectly. The result? Never getting off first base. Just like with exercising and eating right, commit to taking action, do it, and then let it go.

Whenever I suggest an action, whether it's take a walk or work on your refirement plan, women will inevitably say, "It's just one more thing I've got to do. I'm busy caregiving so many other people. I don't have the time." The best advice I've heard about the time issue comes from Governor Huckabee. I was presenting him an award, and he said, "People constantly ask me how I find time to do what I need to. And I say, I don't find the time, I *make* it." You need to make the time to achieve your Financial Fitness.

⇒Fit to Live Essentials⇐

Using your score from the "Are You Financially Fit to Live?" test, you'll continue to build your individual program with the tips below. As in previous chapters, you'll begin according to your current level.

TO SURVIVE:

If you received a score of 0 to 6 on the test, focus your energy here first. Once you've mastered these, feel free to move up to the tips in "To Enjoy."

1. Have the Courageous Conversation

One-third of us have never had an in-depth conversation with our spouse, family, or advisor about how much money we'll need for retirement. And two-thirds of women have not discussed with their partners financial issues relating to health, like life insurance, wills, or long-term care insurance. Most say they are willing to discuss it, but less than half don't initiate the conversation. Courage, people. Yes it's scary to think about the difficult things that might happen. It's like not going to the doctor because you don't want to know the truth about your health. How can you get better if you don't? Same here—the relief you get from having a plan can't be underestimated. Want further proof? Research shows that the happiest folks protect their families and themselves with adequate insurance. Whether you need to talk to yourself or your spouse, it's time to tell your True Truth—you need a refirement plan, you are going to die, and even if you stay in Fit to Live shape, you may become disabled or need long-term care. Acknowledge reality and talk about it with your spouse—or yourself.

2. Write a Will and a Medical Power of Attorney

Now that you've owned up to yourself that you're not going to be around forever, make sure that you get to express your wishes as to where you want your assets to go after your death. That's why you need a will. You also need to make sure you get to express what kind of medical care you want if you can't speak for yourself. The form for a medical power of attorney (also referred to as a living will or an advance directive) varies from state to state. Be sure that you understand what it means. I always advise talking to a lawyer first. If you want to access some basic information about how to start this process, go to www.caringinfo.org. You can also go to www.nolo.com for advice about wills.

3. Get a Refirement Goal

To become Physically Fit to Live, you strive to reach a certain body composition goal. The same holds true for being Financially Fit to Live. You've *got* to know what you'll need. Because everyone's situation is unique, I can't tell you how much to save for refirement (although 15 percent of pretax income per year is a rough rule of thumb these days to have enough to last our whole lives). Go to www.choosetosave.org. It has a retirement calculator (as well as all kinds of other useful calculators, like how much mortgage you can afford and how much you need to save for your kid's college education).

4. Fire Up the Investments

Start investing or, if you have already been, increase it as much as you can. Take advantage of your company's 401k or other plans. Just like you did for your emergency savings, have the money withdrawn directly from your paycheck. You're never going to miss it if you don't get it. If your work doesn't have a plan, there are lots of mutual funds that can be opened with a $50-a-month systematic withdrawal. Start with an amount you feel comfortable with and then increase it every year. Let's say you start saving at 5 percent of your salary because you feel like that's what you can afford. The next time you get a raise, add another percent into your savings. Again, treat investing just like you treat weight reduction—slow and steady.

Don't forget that whatever money you put into your 401k or IRA is pretax, which means by investing, you may lower your taxable income and even drop to a less-steep tax bracket.

LOOKING FOR SPARE MONEY TO INVEST?

✓ Put your tax refund into your 401k or IRA. You've already lived without it.

✓ Wait a year to purchase a new car—if you save $220 a month on payments, that's $2,640 in a year!

✓ Pack your lunch—if you save $5 per workday, that's $100 per month.

✓ How much did you used to spend on snacks, sodas, and specialty coffees a day? Add it up and have that amount automatically deposited each month into your 401k or IRA.

✓ Take a walk instead of shopping—you'll help Mind and Muscle too.

✓ Get a credit card with no annual fee and a low interest rate.

✓ Give gifts of time or make something homemade.

To get lots of other ideas, check out "What's it worth to reduce my spending?" at www.choosetosave.org. It will help you figure out what you can save by making changes like I suggested. For instance, if you can reduce expenses by $7,500 a year and invest that, you'll have over $90,000 in 10 years—and much more by the time you retire.

5. Purchase Protection

Whether you need life, health, disability, or long-term care insurance and how much depends on your situation. For life, consider the following: Is someone dependent on your income besides you? How would they pay off the mortgage without you? Or do all the household tasks? You can check out the life insurance calculator at www.choosetosave.org. To compare prices once you know what you need, check out www.insweb.com. You can get comparisons on health insurance there too.

What if you got hurt? The Insurance Information Institute (www.iii.org) can give you all the particulars on how to think about the important issue of disability insurance, and www.healthdecisions.org lists all the companies that offer these policies. Finally, if you are over 50, seriously consider long-term care insurance. To get started, go to the American Association for Long-Term Care Insurance: www.aaltci.org/consumer.

TO ENJOY:

If you scored a 7 to 13 on the test, just take a quick look at the "To Survive" suggestions. If you feel you have them covered, you can start here.

1. Get a Financial Fitness Trainer (a.k.a. Planner)

Just like you might treat yourself to a personal trainer to get Physically Fit to Live, you might benefit from the help of a financial planner to become Financially Fit to Live. He or she will take a look at your overall financial picture and make recommendations.

How to find a good one? This is a relationship based on trust. Talk to friends, like you would to find a good doctor or hairdresser. My friends at www.prudential.com have a place on their Web site for you to put in your ZIP code and find someone local. The non-profit Financial Planning Association (www.fpanet.org) can also make recommendations in your area. It's smart to interview three people so that you can judge the chemistry between you. Ask for references, what their credentials are, whether they are licensed, whether they have ever been fined or suspended, what their fees are, and whether they recommend a wide variety of products or one company. Finally, ask how they make their money—that will tell you what their stake is and how it might influence their recommendations to you.

> "Retirement at 65 is ridiculous. When I was 65, I still had pimples."
>
> —*George Burns*

2. Learn about Stocks and Bonds

You've got a good financial plan and feel more secure about your refirement future. How about learning more about the world of investments? No, you don't need an MBA. Instead, with the help of the resources we've provided in this section, as well as the guidance from financial planners, you'll be able to increase your knowledge base as well as Financial Fitness. You'll also learn about yourself. Investing is all about risk tolerance—how much risk you are willing to take for what reward. Approach this the way you'd approach learning about new nutritional or physical activity options. The template's the same. It's an enjoyable adventure of discovery.

3. Join the Clued-In Club

When you were first learning about Financial Fitness, I'll bet that if someone showed you the *Wall Street Journal* Money and Investing section, you probably broke out into hives. Well, now that you're past that aversion, how about hanging out with like-minded individuals? Subscribe to newspapers *(Financial Times, Wall Street Journal),* magazines *(Fortune, Entrepreneur),* or stay current with books, television, and radio programs, and Web sites on investing. Doing so will expand your Financial Fitness practices.

TO CHALLENGE:

If you scored a 14 to 20 on the test, just take a quick look at the "To Survive" and "To Enjoy" tips. If you feel you have them covered, you can start here.

1. Get Refired and Give Back

The refirement years present golden opportunities to find ways to use your skill set to give back to humanity. One of my patients, a psychologist, is a perfect example. He indulged his love of travel but with a twist. Everywhere he went, he also found groups in need of psychological support. He would visit them, share his therapeutic skills, and then receive in turn a special gift of cultural sharing and learning. He accomplished all of this while also making the time to take better care of himself. He shed 45 pounds of excess fat, and his waistline fell from a Toxic Belly girth of 44 inches to a healthy 36 inches. You can do this too. Go back to your Power Why and start the adventure.

> "Money is better than poverty, if only for financial reasons."
> —*Woody Allen*

2. Start Your Own Business

Ever wanted to start your own business? Now that you're at the Challenge level, how about investing in that idea and making it a reality? Approach it as you would any other new endeavor—cautiously. Study, assess, and research every aspect of your proposed business concept. Pull together a team to guide and support you. Start lean and mean. One of my patients, a government computer expert, started a Web site business from her home. On top of that, she became an online computer science teacher at a local university. She's joyfully challenged and, working from home and not plagued by long commutes and endless committee meetings, she has plenty of time to work out and prepare healthy meals. Sounds like a Fit to Live life!

3. Do One, A² One, Teach One

If you've gotten to the Challenge level of Financial Fitness, you're sadly in the grand minority of folks out there. You've learned how to A² through your financial life. Ever feel the need to help guide others? Why not join with community and college groups and become an ongoing volunteer and teacher to so many needy men and women out there? The return on investment for you is the satisfaction of knowing you helped someone desperate for your real-world advice pull themselves up out of debt, or guide them to realize a dream—owning a house, starting a business. Moreover, it keeps you flexing your mental muscles.

FIT TO LIVE MONEY PLAN AT A GLANCE

SPENDING	ACCRUING RESERVES	LONG-TERM PLANNING	INVESTING
Tracking cash flow/ creating a budget	Savings	Wills and living wills	Stocks and bonds
Health insurance	Emergency fund	Business succession plan (if applicable)	
Disability insurance		Plan to discuss and explain finances with key family members	
Life insurance		Essential income for survivors	
Long-term care insurance		Get it now since most will need it	

PART 5

Macrocosm: Are You Environmentally Fit to Live?

"This is the true nature of home—it is the place of Peace. . . . "
—*JOHN RUSKIN*

This section addresses the question, Are you Environmentally Fit to Live? To Survive, to Enjoy, to Challenge—and to save your life? Environmental Fitness is all about creating the outer conditions that support your ability to be Fit to Live. A fit environment helps you add more to that precious reserve of Body Dollars you need to maintain your health and wellness. If you can find your treadmill or weight set, you're going to use them, banking more Body Dollars to keep you mentally and physically strong.

You may never have considered how so many factors in our outside world have the potential to stand in the way of permanently cutting the Toxic Belly Fat. In this section, you'll learn what moves you need to make to control your environment rather than allowing it to control you. I'll show you how to keep practicing your A^2 when a wellness-supporting environment becomes toxic. You'll even discover how being Environmentally

Fit can save your life in an emergency. By the time you finish this section, you will have the final piece you need to get and stay Fit to Live—lean, strong, and fearless for life.

To begin, find out your current level of Macrocosm Fitness. Circle the answer that most closely matches your situation:

1. Your running shoes are:
   a. Somewhere in the back of your closet—you think—but everything is so cluttered you're not sure.
   b. Right next to the door.
   c. Either next to the door, or under the bed, or behind the sofa or . . .

2. When you step into your house after coming home from work, you feel:
   a. Calm and relaxed. Your home is a true sanctuary.
   b. Maybe a bit frazzled by kids, dogs, and the crisis du jour, but basically happy to be home.
   c. So overwhelmed by general chaos—dirty dishes, clothes scattered on the floor, etc.—frankly, it's a relief to go to work.

3. While driving to work, your boss calls and asks if you could swing by the airport and pick up an important client. After you hang up, you:
   a. Have to pull off by the side of the road to get rid of all the empty coffee cups, junk-food wrappers, and soda cans that litter the interior.
   b. Dust off the dog's blanket in the airport parking lot, and offer a quick apology to the client when she enters.
   c. Recall that the client is from Denver, and make a note to ask her about her city's great restaurants, museums, and natural attractions.

4. You've just had a very hectic day at the office. When you get home, you find the noise and general chaos level is at red—the television blares, the video games bleep, the kids squabble over who ate the last chocolate-chip cookie. You are most likely to:
   a. Take an aspirin or a glass of wine and get started on dinner.
   b. Inform your family that you need a time-out, and then spend a good 20 minutes decompressing in the part of your home where everyone knows they can't disturb you.

    c. Turn off the electronics and tell your kids that if they aren't quiet, there will be no more cookies, ever.

5. If the health police were to raid your kitchen, they'd:
    a. Award you a good-citizen award after finding your refrigerator and pantry filled with fruits, vegetables, whole grains, and lean proteins.
    b. Issue you a warning for those potato chips and frozen pizzas.
    c. Wrap yellow tape around your cupboard and refrigerator doors, declaring the entire area a health hazard.

6. Your bank calls to say they've noticed an inconsistency on your statement and just want to double-check that no one's stealing your identity. You:
    a. Ask if they can hold the line—you just need a little time to find your statements.
    b. Tell them you'll have to call them back. Finding all your bank records could take half the day.
    c. Grab the folder that contains all your bank statements.

7. A tornado blows through your hometown, knocking out the power. You:
    a. Know exactly where the flashlight, candles, radio, and batteries are.
    b. Would probably find the flashlight—but can't say for sure that the batteries work.
    c. Are sitting in the dark.

8. Your definition of "getting back to nature" is:
    a. Having the hostess seat your party in the garden.
    b. Taking a walk in the park on a regular basis.
    c. Spending at least a week in a secluded place where there are no phones, televisions, or Internet access.

9. How much time do you spend outside?
    a. You walk, run, or bike almost every day, at least in good weather.
    b. Basically none. You commute more than ½ hour, which is why you never get outside during the week and have trouble fitting in the exercise. Or your neighborhood is so unsafe (traffic, violence) that you take your life in your hands to go outside.
    c. You walk, bike, or run outside a couple of times a week.

10. You are exposed to cigarette smoke:

    a. Whenever you take your smoke break.

    b. Whenever you go to a party or your husband lights his cigars.

    c. Hardly ever. You don't smoke and don't really know anyone who does.

Scoring:

For each question, match your answer to the proper score.

1. a, 0; b, 2; c, 1		6. a, 1; b, 0; c, 2
2. a, 2; b, 1; c, 0		7. a, 2; b, 1; c, 0
3. a, 0; b, 1; c, 2		8. a, 0; b, 1; c, 2
4. a, 0; b, 2; c, 1		9. a, 2; b, 0; c, 1
5. a, 2; b, 1; c, 0		10. a, 0; b, 1; c, 2

Add up your scores for the 10 questions and check the key below.

0 to 6: Fit to Survive. Great opportunities could be knocking at your door, but you're so overloaded with clutter that you'll be lucky if you can even find the door. You probably don't think that the state of your car interior or a walk in nature has anything to do with why you're not reaching your fitness goals, but it does! Job one: Clear out the smoke. Even if you don't smoke, when you spend a great deal of time around someone who does, you

---

Bottom-Line Results from Becoming Environmentally Fit to Live to Enjoy

■ You'll cut the clutter enough to save your life in times of crisis and stress.

■ You'll support a lifestyle that allows you to bank extra Body Dollars through healthy living habits.

■ You'll reduce or eliminate the stress overeating associated with a Toxic Living Environment.

■ You'll cut your Toxic Belly Fat and keep it off.

■ You'll cut the Mental Fat of clutter, chaos, and helplessness, replacing it with the clean, open mental and physical spaces to rest, revitalize, and live in wellness.

increase your risk of dying from lung cancer by 20 percent. If that person smokes more than 40 cigarettes a day, your increased risk of dying from lung cancer goes up by 90 percent. A Fit to Live Environment makes it easier to become Fit to Live.

7 to 13: Fit to Enjoy. You are starting to realize the impact that your environment has on your health. Perhaps you cleaned out your closet last weekend and realized that not only do you not miss the puffy-sleeved dresses you wore in college, you have found that the extra space is keeping your head clearer. Most important, you're making your home and living spaces safer and more Fit to Live user-friendly. You're thinking about preventing falls and protecting your precious body from injury and disability. Of the nearly 20,000 deaths and more than 21 million medical visits because of preventable home injuries, falls are by far the number one reason.

14 to 20: Fit to Challenge. You're queen or king of your environment. When you wake up in the morning, you feel in control of your living and working spaces. Your stress level is low because you have created a way of living that is manageable, that allows you to adapt and adjust when challenges occur. You have integrated the outdoors into your life and feel a greater sense of community and connectedness to nature. You're one of the 90 percent of nature-loving people who seek out experiences nature on a regular basis because they create a sense of energy and well-being. You may even be among the 77 percent of people back from a nature retreat who initiated a major life change in their relationship or career as a result. You have energetically blasted the roadblocks—such as a cluttered home, unsafe environment, and toxic (health-destructive) friends— that hold so many people back. Your Environmental Fitness is not just saving you calories and frustration—your preparedness will save your life. You are the Fit to Live champion.

CHAPTER 13

You Can't Take a Walk If You Can't Find Your Sneakers

"The adaptation of individuals to the needs of the body, the community,
and the environment in which they live is mandatory for survival."
—ERIK ERIKSON

I s your home or workspace Fit to Live in? Do you have miles of piles all over the place? This chapter is a wake-up call to how the environmental fat you're hauling around day after day is landing on your waistline. Becoming Fit to Live is not just about eating well and getting in the exercise. You need an environment to live and work in that is conducive to practicing your healthy living habits. You can't take a walk if you can't find your sneakers. You can't eat well if your fridge and cabinets are filled with food that is junk, outdated, or nonexistent because you haven't been to the store. You can't live cost effectively when you can't find your checkbook or bills to pay on time, because they've been thrown somewhere on the desk from hell. How can you feel calm and peaceful when you're walking around in angst, shame, and guilt, surrounded by chaos?

Messy living and working spaces lead to distressed minds, which lead to Toxic Lifestyle habits like overeating and overdrinking, which lead to more Toxic Belly Fat. Cluttered environment, cluttered belly. Make that connection, and you'll create a Power Why that will help you stay focused enough to become Environmentally Fit to Live.

Just like we've ballooned physically, so have we done in our home environments. We're not only mindlessly eating too much food, we're bingeing on too much stuff. Our mountains of possessions and the clutter that results are a huge energy drain on our Mind, Mouth, Muscle, and Money.

"What's the big deal?" you ask. Well, believe it or not, the bigger you are, the more stuff you probably have lying around. I discovered this while filming the National Body Challenge for Discovery Health TV. I went into people's homes and tripped over clutter everywhere. Garages were scary places where that bike or weight set was buried under tons of Christmas tree lights, broken appliances, and deflated basketballs.

I vividly recall the times when my patients finally make the Mouth-Mess Connection. They sit before me in wonderment recalling how they mysteriously have begun to clean up everything from the banana peels and fast-food wrappers in the back of the car to hallway closets with all those boxes and clothes. I smile and congratulate them. Instead of dropping into a food coma in front of the tube, they're now more aware of how toxic their living space is and how it fosters their distress, overeating, and Toxic Lifestyle habits. They begin naturally gravitating to the clean, open spaces where Environmental Fitness can begin.

⇒Our Toxic Lifestyle⇐
Mountains of Too Much

"Our houses are such unwieldy property that we are often imprisoned rather than housed in them."
—HENRY DAVID THOREAU

For centuries as cave dwellers, our possessions were limited to what we could carry. Clutter didn't support survival. (Running from a saber-tooth while hauling a TV, CD player, Crackberry, cell phone, makeup bag, and laptop computer would not portend well for your life span.) Once we settled down on farms and in cities, we lived in simple, functional dwellings and worked hard to provide the basics.

> "If you can organize your
> kitchen, you can organize
> your life."
> —*Louis Parrish*

As with food, our goals with possessions and homes were with having enough, not too much. Dwellings were tiny, just as they are in many third world countries today—about 500 square feet. Possessions were limited to a few cooking pots, baskets, and wash basins, one or two sets of clothes, and a bed where frequently, the whole family slept.

Slowly, over time, as we in the developed world became more prosperous, our homes grew. So did the stuff inside them. And so did we. Fifty years ago, the average American kitchen measured about 80 square feet, and the average American man weighed 166 pounds. Today, the average American kitchen measures about 225 square feet, and the average American man weighs about 191 pounds. During this same time, men's waistlines exploded from a 32-inch girth to one that's pushing 40 inches. Could there be a connection?

Look around your home. I'll bet at some point in your life, often inspired by a long-forgotten New Year's resolution, you went on a wellness binge and bought exercise equipment. You know, an ab roller, stationary bike, or treadmill. Eventually, they became expensive clothes hangers. We try to ignore them. And when we do experience a brief wake-up from our mind-body dissociation, we feel guilt for having gone to all the effort and expense to buy these heaps of metal, only to feel like we've failed once again in the almighty quest for the healthy, fit body.

Feel overwhelmed by the miles of piles? When you stumble into your home after work and hopelessly gaze at the mess in every room, do you feel that sinking feeling of helplessness, shame, and defeat? If this is your mindset, you're stirring up those stress

Fascinating FAToid

The Fridge/Fat Connection

The average size of refrigerators increased by 10 percent since 1972 and so also the number of fridges per home. Good grief. **Bottom line:** We got seduced by the "bigger is better" ads. It's time to connect the dots—oversize fridges, oversize food containers, mindless eating, and Toxic Belly Fat. Time to bag the bigger trends if we ever want to cut the fat from our environment and our bodies.

Fascinating FAToid
Gain More Time for Life

Cleaning experts say that ridding your home of clutter will cut down on your housework by 40 percent. **Bottom line:** The real reward for keeping a decluttered environment is the ability to spend more joyful time with yourself and your loved ones.

hormones I told you about in Mind. You go from zero to anxiety, walk past the mess, and head for the kitchen where the supersized fridge and kitchen cabinets overloaded with anesthetics await you. Back into food coma you go, and you're wearing that stress and extra food as Toxic Belly Fat.

Our goal with decluttering is to create a home and workspace that lays down the red carpet for your Fit to Live life. It may even save your life someday. Want proof? One day, one of my regular patients came to me with quite a story. Late at night, she heard noises in her basement. Living alone, she was terrified. She called 911, but as the footsteps began to ascend the stairs, she dropped the phone and ran to her bedroom drawer where she kept a heavy-duty flashlight. Grasping it tightly, she waited for the perpetrator to come into the room, and then, with all her strength, she clocked him on the head. He dropped, she hopped over him and, running fast, made it out the door onto her lawn, where she screamed as loudly as she could. By then, the police had arrived, and the burglar was apprehended.

When I first met this woman, she was depressed and disorganized, overweight with Toxic Belly Fat, dragged down by the Mental Fat of fear of life's stresses. Two years later, she became the heroine of her own story. How? She took herself on, cut through her Mental Fat, and with dogged determination became Fit to Live. She cleaned up the clutter in her living spaces and organized her possessions so she knew where to go in an emergency. She had a special place in an extra room she devoted to her weight lifting—just a mat, some tubing, and hand weights. She walked outdoors most days, keeping her sneakers by the front door. So when the crime occurred, she was Fit to Live to survive the crisis. There was no stumbling over clutter or panicking about where the flashlight was. Physically, she was strong and ready to take him on. Mentally, she was ready to fight for her life. She had achieved the ultimate Fit to Live goal—to become lean, strong, and fearless. That's what I want for you too.

⇒Fit to Live⇐
A Home That Supports Your Fitness

"Your mind, which is yourself, can be likened to a house. The first necessary move then is to rid that house of all but furnishings essential to success."
—JOHN MCDON

I first began to understand the relationship between body weight and environmental weight from a patient. "You know," she said one day, "in the past, I would have just sat on the couch mindlessly eating in front of the tube. But the better I feel about myself, the more I have the urge to purge all my piles. Plus, cleaning out my closets is good exercise—and it gives me something else to do besides eat!"

I started to talk to other patients about decluttering and discovered that as they awakened from the dissociative trance they were in, they awakened not only to their body weight, but also to their closet weight, their desk weight, their attic and basement weight. Suddenly, the guys were in the garage, organizing and decluttering. Women found themselves hunting through the closets and doing redecorating. Before they were in food comas;

Voice of Success: Catching the Decluttering Bug

Jeniffer White removed 37 pounds; husband Jeff removed over 125 pounds

"Everything in our house was a mess. Jeff and I were overweight and lazy. We cleaned, but never felt motivated to dejunk. I had brand-new tennis shoes in the closet that I'd never worn, but I could find only one. We had gym equipment in the garage covered with boxes. When we started to get fit, we realized we had to have the exercise stuff in our face. Because if you can't see it, you don't think about it. We began to clean up everything. It felt so good to accomplish something. We decluttered the whole house and redid the backyard. Accomplishing the decluttering helped us stay motivated to change everything else—eating habits and exercise—because when you have one success, you feel more successful all the way around."

consumed with hopelessness and lack of motivation, they didn't feel good or fit enough to make environmental changes. As they got fitter in Mind, Mouth, Muscle,

> "A large part of virtue consists in good habits."
> —*William Paley*

and Money, they also created time and energy to optimize their living spaces.

I thought I was the only person who understood this relationship between clutter and Toxic Belly Fat. Then recently, I was having dinner with a new colleague of mine from Discovery Health: Dan Ho. Dan's the author of *Rescue from Domestic Perfection* and host of *The Dan Ho Show* about how to simplify your home life. He's also removed 120 pounds of Toxic Body Fat. When I began talking to him about the fat/clutter connection, he said, "I may have lost over 100 pounds, but I dropped five times that much decluttering my house."

As Dan discovered, a crucial aspect of being Fit to Live is about creating a lighter home environment that supports your new healthy lifestyle. As you contemplate these important changes, consider my bottom-line suggestions.

THE FIVE FIT TO LIVE DECLUTTERING PRINCIPLES

1. Your External Environment Is a Reflection of Your Internal Environment

People usually are fairly consistent when it comes to neatness or messiness. Alright, everyone's allowed that one spot in their home that looks like hell. But for all intents and purposes, there's usually a direct parallel between how you take care of your environment and how you take care of yourself.

Right now, go to your car and take a look. What do you see? Dust and dirt inside and out? The floor littered with soda cans and snack wrappers and apple cores from 4 weeks ago? If the way your car looks was a message to you about your life, what would the message be? Here's what some patients of mine said their cars expressed: "Shabby, sloppy, uncared for." "Like I don't care." "A junk-food wrapper tornado just blew through."

Is your car reflecting how you feel about yourself? A tidy Macrocosm goes with a tidy Mind and Body. That's why my "To Survive" recommendations at the end of the chapter include one decluttering task for each M. Believe me, doing these five things will make it *so* much easier to become Fit to Live all around.

2. Your Home Should Support Your Power Why

Remember again your Power Why and that what you said gives you joy in the Mind section. Now look at your home. Does it reflect what you say is most precious to you? You say you love to journal. But your desk is piled high with magazines you've been trying for 3 years to read so there's no place to write, and your journal hasn't been seen since 1999. You say television isn't important to you; why do you own 23 of them? Organize to be able to enjoy what really matters to you in your life—time with family and friends, gardening, writing that novel—whatever gives you meaning and joy.

3. Think of Carrot Cake When It Comes to Decluttering

When you're trimming closet fat, treat it like eating carrot cake. Take small slices. If you try to do the entire house in 1 hour, you'll just end up with a bigger mess—with the Mental Fat of discouragement and hopelessness as well. Slice it off one spot at a time—your desk, one closet, the living room, one set of cabinets. Just like I've been saying with the four other Ms, it's very important that you take a little patience pill here and aim to achieve small steps.

YOUR CLOSETS, YOUR SELF

Look at your working space at home and at the office. Do you see a pattern? Here are some common ones:

1. Cram it all into drawers that are too full to open and pretend everything's okay.
2. Cover every available surface and make walkways through the junk.
3. Surrender to the mess and never invite anyone over.
4. Chaos broken up by occasional mad cleanups for company.

Now look at yourself in the mirror. Notice any parallels? Denial and dissociation like #1? Camouflaging your Toxic Belly Fat under hide-it clothes and ignoring the fat as well as the high cholesterol, high blood pressure, and blood sugar too? Giving up and not even trying like #2 and #3? Crash dieting before key occasions, then back to the unfit Mouth and Muscle habits like #4? Use the skills you've learned in the other 4Ms to take yourself on and get Environmentally Fit here too.

Fascinating FAToid

Reclaim 2 Days a Year While Decluttering

The average person gets 30 pounds of junk mail per year. With one quick visit to www. dmaconsumers.org/offmailinglist.html, you can stop this clutter from coming to your door. If you spend 10 minutes a day looking at catalogs, getting rid of junk mail will give you 52 more hours every single year. Not to mention eliminating all those piles and saving all kinds of trees! **Bottom line:** Get to your computer for this important piece of decluttering.

Approach it with a plan. Be methodical and prioritize. Go first for those things that will directly affect your ability to become Fit to Live in the other 4Ms. Dig in the bottom of that closet. I know you've got sneakers in there somewhere. Find them so you can walk regularly. Next the socks, then the sweats, and then the other piece to your CD player, and you're ready to rock.

Do not wing this. That's part of what got you into trouble in the first place. Establish organizing rituals. For instance, say to yourself, "Every Saturday morning, I'll go through all the newspapers I left in a huge gigantic heap all week. I will blast through them and put them in recycling as fast as possible so I have nothing left." Ritual is so important in self-care whether you're ritualizing shopping for food or decluttering. You can even combine rituals. For instance, Saturday morning, as soon as you come home from grocery shopping and before you put the groceries away is the perfect time to clean the refrigerator or the next kitchen cabinet.

If you have a problem decluttering, get help. There are software programs, books, and people to assist you. Go to www.drpeeke.com and follow the links under Macrocosm to find a variety of decluttering resources.

4. Use the 12-Month Rule: If You Haven't Used It, Pitch It

If you're not using it now or will definitely not use it within 12 months, get rid of it. (Exception: financial records and receipts for the IRS, which must be kept for 7 years, and other important papers.) Sell it on e-Bay, toss it out. Or best of all, give it away to people, groups, or facilities in need, such as Goodwill or Salvation Army.

This is particularly important if your closet looks like Filene's Basement on a bad day. You know what I mean—full of 33 different sizes because of the roller coaster you've been on

> ## DO A DAILY 10-MINUTE TIDY
>
> Do you keep waiting for that free weekend to tackle your overflowing guest bedroom closet? Instead, take 10 minutes in the morning or evening and knock off a piece of it. Organize the gift wrap one day, the recycling bins another. Just like successful weight removers look for times during the day for physical activity, finding 10 minutes to tidy will actually get you somewhere rather than waiting for that mythical big block of time to materialize.

with your body. I want you to signal to yourself that you're permanently removing Toxic Belly Fat by giving away your "fat" clothes as soon as they become too big for you. Don't wait 12 months, 12 hours, or even 12 minutes. Out with the oversize belts, slacks, T-shirts, tent dresses, and elastic-waist pants. Your weight is going down, not up!

5. Be Consistent, Not Perfect

Alright, maybe you've decluttered your home space, but your workspace looks like a bomb just hit it. Be consistent across the board, and remove attic weight, basement weight, bookshelf weight, car weight.

As you go about cutting your Environmental Fat, be very clear about one thing: I am *not* giving you permission to become obsessed with perfection. You're not going for spotless, just workable. Remember—perfection isn't possible. This is a living, breathing, dynamic process. It's part of your life journey. Don't waste your precious life trying to meet some impossible standard. All you're trying to do is create space that helps you be Fit to Live, not win the Homemaker of the Century award. Save the time and energy you would put into rolling the hand towels for taking that walk or biking with your kids.

⇒Fit to Live Essentials⇐

Using your score from the "Are You Environmentally Fit to Live?" test, you'll continue to build your individual program with the tips below. As in previous chapters, you'll begin according to your current level.

TO SURVIVE:

If you received a score of 0 to 6 on the test, focus your energy here first. Once you've mastered these, feel free to move up to the tips in "To Enjoy."

1. Mind: Create a Sacred Space for Your Mini-Chills

We all need a spot to restore and renew. Where we look at our lives and think about where, when, and how to A^2. Or just allow our minds to wander and our bodies to chill. It doesn't have to be a fancy meditation room. It could be a big rock in your backyard or a special stuffed chair in a quiet corner. It could be your bathtub. Make sure that you create such a space and include in it whatever elements you want to enhance its restorative abilities—flowers, candles, inspirational quotes, and so on.

And here's the deal. If you live, like so many people, in a circus of family members invading your space, you need to be very assertive about boundaries. That means when you say you're going to your special spot, you don't wish to be disturbed unless it's a life-threatening situation. If you don't fight for the right to have this space and time for yourself, it's not going to happen. Be patient with the folks you live with, since you've probably never established these boundaries before. They got used to your expected "yes" to everyone, anytime. In time, they'll see you mean business. Your Fit to Live business.

2. Mouth: Detoxify Your Food Supply

March into your kitchen right now. Does your fruit bowl have real fruit in it or dust? Bravely and courageously go through every shelf in your fridge. If whatever you're finding does not support the supply or preparation of whole fruits, vegetables, whole grains, or lean protein, toss it. Use the principles from Chapters 4 and 6 as your guides. Keep

Fascinating FATroid

Stop Closet Denial

Sixty percent of those surveyed say they haven't seen the back of their closet in months. Hmmm, there's that 60 percent again—about the same number of us who are overweight or obese. **Bottom line:** Make the Mouth-Mess connection.

asking yourself, "Will this food make me Nutritionally Fit to Live?" If the answer is no, into the garbage or giveaway box it goes. Out of sight, out of mouth. Read the labels and throw out (or give to a food bank if you feel too guilty about wasting food) that high-fat, loaded-with-sugar junk food. Pitch anything that says it has trans fat. Then restock with all those fabulous fruits and veggies (frozen and fresh), whole grains, lean proteins, some healthy nonbingeable treats and Portable Normals you learned about. That way, when you're hungry, you'll *have* to reach for something that will enhance your ability to be Fit to Live.

3. Muscle: Move and Groove at Home and Work

Remember that sacred place in #1? Well, that same principle applies to a sacred place to do the wonderful sculpting and stretching I showed you in the Muscle section. All you need is a mat, and you're in business. You might want to place it in front of the TV, so you can watch an exercise video and to provide entertainment as you work out. When you create a special movement place, you signal to yourself your humble acceptance of regular physical activity in your life. Don't forget to put your sneakers by the door. And keep a packed gym bag in the car. You're answering the call to arms and legs with a commitment of space—your living space.

4. Money: Find a Place for Papers

You may have done a good job getting your financial house in order—stopped the out-of-control spending, started retirement savings, and gotten the insurance you need to support your Fit to Live life. But how about all the documents generated from these changes? Where are your receipts for the IRS? Your bank and credit card statements? Organize your financial paperwork so that you will know where documents are when you need them. You can't track your credit card spending if you have no idea what pile your statement is in.

Your filing system doesn't need to be fancy. In fact, the more complicated the system, the less likely you will be to stick to it. Think nouns—tax receipts, credit card statements, 401ks, etc. With programs like Quicken and online banking, your paper trail may be quite small. However you keep track, you need a place to do it: a desk or table devoted to your computer and a filing cabinet for those papers. If you suffer from chronic paper disorganization, enlist a friend, relative, or professional to help you create a simple system and to get the backlog taken care of. Then all you will have to do is keep up.

5. Macrocosm: Declutter Regularly

Have you ever noticed that, just like two rabbits, clutter has the tendency to reproduce rapidly? You cleaned out the bathroom cabinet only last month, and now you can't open it without a hair dryer and four toilet paper rolls spilling out. Decluttering is not something you do once. Rather, it needs to be a regular part of your Fit to Live lifestyle. Just like Cutting Mental Fat, removing your Toxic Belly Fat, becoming stronger and fitter, and getting your act together financially, you have to do the same with your living and working spaces. As with the other Fit to Live elements, just humbly accept the regular rituals of maintenance.

The good news though, folks, is the more you make Environmental Fitness part of your lifestyle, you won't have a repeat of the piles-of-junk nightmare you had to cope with when you began to awaken from your unfit trance. The Body Dollars you invested the first time around in getting organized will pay off later in dividends of ongoing decluttering ease.

TO ENJOY:

If you scored a 7 to 13 on the test, just take a quick look at the "To Survive" suggestions. If you feel you have them covered, you can start here.

1. Bag the Shame and Embrace Your Power

One of the greatest problems in getting Fit to Live in any M is the shame and guilt that consumes us when we realize the pickle we're in. You know the inner dialogue—"How could I have allowed this to happen?" "What kind of loser am I that I can't even keep up with cleaning my own house?" This negative self-talk consumes huge amounts of Body Dollars. This is especially applicable to women who are the consummate perfectionists and ruminators. Bag the bad talk in your head. Instead, take a deep breath, smile inwardly and outwardly, and seize this very moment to walk into that one scary, messy room with a plan to patiently clean it up. For every pound of clutter you trash, you cut 20 pounds of Mental Fat, which leads to cutting 10 pounds of Body Fat. Feel how much lighter and freer and more joyful you are now?

2. Redo Your Spaces

Feel like doing something new and special to celebrate becoming Environmentally Fit to Live? How about painting your kitchen or sacred space with a color that makes you feel terrific? Got a few Bank Dollars to spare because you're more Financially Fit? How about redoing your kitchen, creating a workout space, or making a plan to open up more spaces throughout your home? Or purchase colorful and fun containers and file cabinets and organize your papers and possessions. What about a sound system with calming music or a bubbling water fountain for your bedroom? Fresh flowers are a gift to your senses, and muted lighting nurtures a peaceful environment. The options are endless when you seek joy as you become Environmentally Fit to Live.

3. Get a Buddy or Two on Board

Talk with whomever you're living with about your newfound goals. Get their support not only for the technical environmental changes you want to make, but to help you protect the self-time you need in your sacred place. Sharing like this is integral to building the Body Dollar reserves that can weather life's stresses. Can you team up and paint some rooms together? Can everyone get involved with the kitchen redo? Get help from family and/or friends to clean out the cupboards. Shop together for healthy food. What about taking on the garage as a family project and celebrating each time you decluttered by going to the movies or making a terrific family meal together? Teaming on Environmental Fitness is an essential element of the Fit to Live lifestyle.

TO CHALLENGE:

If you scored a 14 to 20 on the test, just take a quick look at the "To Survive" and "To Enjoy" tips. If you feel you have them covered, you can start here.

1. Give Feng Shui a Whirl

Have you ever heard of feng shui? That's the ancient Chinese practice of arrangement to create harmony with nature and good flow of the life force energy or chi (pronounced "chee") in your living space. It's the rage in most lifestyle magazines. There are even feng shui consultants who will come into your home and help you organize your living space. Here are some feng shui ideas to intrigue you:

Food represents wealth to the Chinese, and therefore kitchens generate general happiness. According to feng shui practitioners, chi should flow freely through your home, coming through the front door and leaving out the back. Any clutter, sharp angles, nooks and crannies, and storage areas can slow down energy, causing it to stagnate and become unhealthful. Curious? Go to www.wofs.com to learn more.

2. Emergency-Proof Your Environment

It's not enough to be physically and mentally strong to save your life. You need a living environment that can also help you save your life in case of emergency. Have a police and fire safety expert come in and give you tips about how to keep your home safe. Most will recommend some kind of alarm system, and of course, you must have fire detectors. Know where your flashlights, candles, and matches are located. Keep extra food, water, and medical supplies updated just in case. We live in a post-Katrina, post-9/11 world. Staying in good shape and living in a more secure environment are two factors that may prove to be lifesaving one day.

CHAPTER 14

A Chronic Case of Nature Deficiency

"What is the use of a house if you haven't got a tolerable planet to put it on?"
—HENRY DAVID THOREAU

Nature deficiency is something I discovered when I began to conduct my Peeke Week Retreats in nature, hoping to give people an opportunity to learn just how Mentally and Physically Fit to Live they were. Outside of diehard outdoor athletes, the people with lots of Toxic Belly Fat were amazed at just how out of shape they were, covered in sweat as they scampered over rocks, hoofing it on hiking trails, or gasping for breath as they trudged up each hill. The difference between the groups was that the Fit to Live people had the Body Dollar reserves to hit the hills and keep pace without collapsing. They were able to put their Physical and Mental Fitness to the test with natural challenges. The other group, who thought they were okay, found out that, when placed in nature outside of their usual comfort zone and asked to push beyond it, they had few reserves to succeed. Each group had quite a humbling but exhilarating learning experience.

When was the last time you were out in nature? How did it make you feel? This chapter explores the transition from green place to cement place and what that's done to our well-being and our waists. We'll look at how to infuse some healthy green and detox our surroundings, as well as explore why we need tree therapy, so we can become truly Environmentally Fit to Live.

⇒Our Toxic Lifestyle⇐
Nature, What's Nature?

"When a man moves away from nature, his heart becomes hard."
—LAKOTA PROVERB

Nature has come full circle. In the beginning, of course, the out of doors was our home. We used all our senses—sight, smell, touch, taste, hearing—not only to survive, but also to thrive within the natural world. As we moved from caves to farms, we still stayed tied to the daily and yearly cycles of nature. Some folks lived in cities, but very few. In 1790, only 5 percent of the US population were city dwellers; the rest lived in rural areas. Slowly over the next 150 years, we began deserting the farms for cities and suburbs. But even up to the 1970s, most of us lived closer to nature than we do now.

Now we seem to be coming back to our roots. People are paying extra money to have a larger green space around their homes; to locate in places close to walking, biking, and hiking trails; and to revel in all that is natural. New books show us how to build homes with a seamless inside and outside connection—rooms and decks built around trees, huge windows to give the sense of living under the sun and natural surroundings.

Are you old enough to remember walking to school and playing outside on weekends and after school? As we explored in the last chapter, homes used to be small, and backyards were big. I had a typical childhood in the late '50s and '60s in suburban northern California. When I came home from school, I got a quick graham cracker and apple snack and then I was outside to terrorize the neighborhood with my friends. We lived across the street from the beach and one block from the zoo. When I wasn't at one of those two places, my friends and I played in undeveloped fields and woods, as well as one another's big backyards. I was in seventh heaven.

Then, between the 1970s and 2006, the US population grew by almost 100 million. These days, 80 percent of Americans live in urban areas—cities or the sprawling suburbs that surround them. Because of this spreading, we all live in our cars, which makes it a bit hard to experience nature except as a blur going by. Today, only 16 percent of us live close enough not to drive to work; in the '60s, that number was over 30 percent. Once we finally arrive at the office after fighting freeway gridlock, we are crammed into tiny offices and cubicles, often with no windows and no access to open space at all.

When we struggle home in the evenings, we unlock the front door and collapse on the couch for the duration of the evening. How much time do you spend outdoors a day? If you do dare walk around your neighborhood, do you ever see anyone out in their front yard? Or on the sidewalks? We're all holed up inside, with our gigantic refrigerators and oversize reclining chairs. We now spend 90 percent of our time indoors. Ninety percent!

Many of us want this to be different. A major national study found that a majority of Americans would like to walk and bike more rather than drive. But many neighborhoods don't even have sidewalks that would encourage walking, and some neighborhoods are simply unsafe to walk in.

Where we live, say experts, is one of the most important determinants of whether we exercise. Things such as lack of sidewalks, hills, heavy traffic, roaming dogs, a dearth of scenery, and high levels of crime all keep us from moving. So do long distances between homes, malls, and schools in suburbs. Adults who live in houses built before 1973 are significantly more likely to walk 1 mile or farther more than 20 times a month than those who live in newer houses, regardless of race, gender, age, income, or health-related problems. How come? Sidewalks. Our newer neighborhoods have been designed around our sedentary, car-based toxic lifestyle.

CARS ARE TOXIC TO OUR WAISTLINES

Did you know that every hour you spend in the car means a 6 percent rise in your risk for obesity? Yikes! There's also brand-new evidence that if you spend more than 40 minutes a day in the car, you lose 1.25 hours of sleep—and an additional 15 minutes of sleep for every 8 minutes driving. Remember, lack of sleep shows up around your waistline. So hop out of your car and into your sneakers.

Fascinating FAToid

Life Span by ZIP Code

Where you live has profound implications on *how long* you live—as much as 35 years! It's not due only to income or access to medical care, say researchers, but also shared customs and norms regarding diet, exercise, smoking, and alcohol consumption. **Bottom line:** You are influenced—for better or worse—by your surroundings. If you're being negatively affected, take yourself on and put healthy changes into action.

I've been interested in the connection between health and the environment since I was a college student. I was premed and did a second major in conservation of natural resources. I discovered with shock and horror the "big disconnect." On one side of the campus, my professors were extolling the virtues of healthy living to prevent disease. But directly across campus, students in the City and Regional Planning program were learning how to cram homes together to squeeze optimal cost-effectiveness from every square inch of terrain. So we're supposed to maintain good health and well-being living in cement blocks with few parks, sidewalks, and home gardens.

My concern was part of the reason I entered the UC Berkeley's School of Public Health for my masters' degree. That was years ago. Now my fear has come to haunt us all in the worst way, because it's all fine and dandy for me to say, "Go take a walk." But if you have nowhere safe or accessible to walk, what are you supposed to do?

I had a big lesson in this while taping a show for the National Body Challenge. One of my families, the Holmeses, lived in a modest home in southeast Los Angeles, in an area of drive-by shootings and drug trafficking. One very hot day, my producer said, "Dr. Peeke, it's time for you and the Holmeses to go for a walk for the camera."

As I was happily tightening up my sneakers, the head of the household, Shequestra Holmes, said, "Well, now, walking in this neighborhood could be a bit challenging."

I said, "I realize it's a little hot today. But you've got plenty of sidewalks."

"No, no, no," she replied. "We don't even walk our dog in this neighborhood. The pit bulls and rottweilers roam free, so there are packs of wild dogs in the neighborhood looking for trouble. That's why we have a golf club by the front door, in case a dog tries to attack us as we go in and out."

By this time, it was 97 degrees in Los Angeles. But it was 150 degrees in my body. Believe me, that was the fastest walking segment I've ever done. My heart broke for this beautiful family whose lives were in peril every time they stepped outside the door. Despite this challenge, the whole family did so well, they were profiled on my show.

Safety issues also mean that kids can't stomp through the snow by themselves to get to school or to roam the neighborhood when they come home. Check this out—in 1977, kids ages 5 to 15 walked or rode their bikes for over 15 percent of their trips. Guess what the number was in 1995? Under 10 percent, a drop of 37 percent. It's just not safe—in terms

A FEW WORDS ABOUT SMOKING

You think smoking is going away? Wrong. A Centers for Disease Control and Prevention survey found that 44.5 million adults and one in four teens are smokers, with Asian American adults and teens and African American teens at a higher rate than other groups. And cigarettes are more toxic now. Nicotine levels in cigarettes have risen 10 percent on average in the past 6 years, making it easier to be addicted and, unfortunately, harder to quit. If you smoke:

✓ You have increased risk of many cancers: lung, lip, pharynx, oral cavity, esophagus, pancreas, voice box, uterus, bladder, and kidney.

✓ You have up to four times the risk of heart disease, 10 times the risk of peripheral vascular disease (narrowing of blood vessels), and double the risk of stroke.

✓ If you're female, you have an increased risk of infertility, premature births, stillbirths, low-birth-weight babies, and sudden infant death syndrome (SIDS). If you're postmenopausal, you'll likely have lower bone density and increased risk of hip fracture.

✓ If you smoke and drink, it's recently been discovered that smokers need to drink more alcohol to get a buzz because nicotine reduces blood alcohol levels. This leads to smokers drinking more, which leads to a buildup of more Toxic Belly Fat.

So if you're smoking now, get off the stuff. If you live with a smoker, help them get off, or get them out of the house when they smoke.

of traffic, stranger danger, and random violence.

Given the dangers, we might as well stay cooped up inside, right? Wrong. Getting outside is one of the best things you can do

> "In all things of nature, there is something of the marvelous."
> —*Aristotle*

to get rid of your Toxic Belly Fat. Science shows there is a direct relationship between access to the outdoors and the size of our bodies. Those who live where they can bike, walk, or take public transit are slimmer and more fit than those who don't. And people who live in counties where homes are spread apart and far from shopping (that old sprawl thing), walk less and weigh more than others.

In fact, the odds you'll be obese rise 10 percent with every 50-point degree of sprawl your home is on the sprawl index. Sprawling counties are spread-out areas where homes are far away from other destinations (like offices and stores), which are generally only accessed by highways where it is dangerous to walk or bike. And guess what? There's even a strong relationship between high blood pressure and greater sprawl. How come? People in sprawling counties walk less for exercise. But they also walk less for errands because there is nowhere for them to go. Distance from recreational facilities, feeling unsafe from crime and traffic, and unattractive neighborhoods are all linked to obesity. So is living in a very isolated area with no access to stores, churches, or schools—nothing to do but eat.

One study of national park attendance found that it grew steadily from the 1930s to 1987 but has dropped by 25 percent since then. What's causing the drop? Over 97 percent of it can be directly attributed to increased screen time—movies, video games, TV, and the Internet. In other words, we're too busy watching nature programs to get up off our rear ends and get out there and interact with the real thing.

Being Environmentally Fit to Live includes other factors besides access to nature. It also includes minimizing the chemicals we're exposed to in our homes from air fresheners, toilet bowl cleaners, mothballs, and other deodorizing products. And what about the biggest indoor polluter of all? Yep. Cigarette smoke.

When we want to become Fit to Live, the environment is a key to helping us achieve our goal. This includes the physical structures we live and work in, the air we breathe, the amount of light we're exposed to, the noise, the smells, and the visual stimuli we experience each day.

⇒Fit to Live⇐
They Don't Call It the Great Outdoors for Nothing

"You are a product of your environment. Choose the environment that will best develop you toward your objective. Analyze your life in terms of its environment. Are the things around you helping you toward success—or are they holding you back?"
—CLEMENT STONE

Regardless where you live and work, each of us has the power to make enough changes to save our lives from the consequences of a toxic environment. While you're cleaning up your external environment, you'll be optimizing your internal self as well. You'll look better as you Cut the Toxic Belly Fat and feel more energized as you Cut the Mental Fat. You've become the lean, strong, and fearless person you deserve to be.

THE FIVE ENVIRONMENTALLY FIT TO LIVE PRINCIPLES

1. A² the Green Way

We all have a deep connection to the natural world. In the past 10 years, there has been such an explosion of understanding of the relationship between our mental health and nature that a new movement, called ecopsychology, has emerged to explore this connection. Ecopsychologists claim we are emotionally bonded to the earth and that the eco-

Fascinating FAToid
Beware the Belly/Smoking Connection

Think smoking will help you lose weight? Research on teenage girls found that smokers and nonsmokers gained at exactly the same rate. Plus, in adults, smoking increases your risk for Toxic Belly Fat, as well as Toxic Belly Fat Syndrome. And the risk rises progressively with the number of cigarettes you smoke. **Bottom line:** Remember what you learned in Chapter 1? It's that inner fat that shortens your life. Another good reason to quit.

Fascinating FAToid

Nature Is Truly Healing

Participating in community gardens helped mental patients eat more healthfully, get more physical activity, and feel greater pride, self-worth, sense of hope, and connection to others. It had similar effects on studies of older people. Even walking through the woods has been shown to rejuvenate and inspire folks of all ages. **Bottom line:** Let nature work its magic on your Mind, Mouth, and Muscle.

logical health of the planet is tied to our own mental health. Nature itself is healing to our minds, bodies, and spirits; it's the perfect playpen for learning how to A^2 to life's stresses.

Here's one example of nature's healing power: People who were surrounded by green space in a Chicago public housing project had better relationships with their neighbors and less domestic violence. Other researchers have found a strong relationship between contact with nature and a sense of well-being and have suggested that being exposed to the natural world be used to help prevent depression and other mental illnesses. Better living through Mother Nature!

People who are Environmentally Fit to Live find ways to get out and experience the mind-body-spiritual connection with nature on a regular basis: A walk in the park at noon, a hike with the family on the weekend, an adventure vacation in the mountains. In nature, we reconnect to all our senses. You don't have your Crackberry, cell phones aren't going off, you don't have 20 things vying for your attention. Just you and the sounds, smells, and sights of nature.

I remember meeting Art Levitt, the head of the US Securities and Exchange Commission, once. He told me he had done Outward Bound over 20 times because it was one of the few times in his life when he was able to have his mind and body focus on one thing. Nobody was asking him for any futures on interest rates. Instead, it was his mind and body. Could he get up that hill? Could he hike that mountain? Could he get around that boulder?

You don't have to become a woodsman to appreciate the out of doors as a place of wonderment, as a place of connectivity with all that is alive. Nature humbles us to the fact that we're just a piece of the action here, that we're not some controlling entity. That perspective can help you understand that you, like all the creatures out there, are just finding ways to survive, to nourish yourself, to A^2. Want to Cut your Mental and Belly Fat? Take a hike!

2. Choose Your Environment Wisely

When I talk about environment, I'm not talking only about the natural world, but also how your senses and health are affected by the places you spend your days and nights. That means what you see, hear, and feel, what you smell and touch, and who you surround yourself with. Brand-new science shows that our brains are actually shaped by the people we spend our time with. Recognize that all these elements are having an effect on you, and start to be conscious about the choices you're making about where to be and whom to be with. You want to spend your time in situations and with people that bring out the best in you and support your Mind, Mouth, Muscle, and Money Fitness.

For instance, are you someone who just thrives on light, yet everywhere you are is dark, and it contributes to feeling hopeless and depressed? Do you listen to soothing music in your car? Or are you tuned to talk radio that's making you anxious and upset? Are you around grumblers and complainers all the time who distress you and send you running to the fridge?

This is about choices. You have to realize the power of your choices. Choose happier, positive people to hang out with. Do the work to find them. Choose to walk in the park with friends, to garden with the family, to paint your walls a bright yellow, or to tell someone you're not going in their car if they smoke. This is the Fit to Live attitude that will save your life.

Voice of Success: "I Can Do Anything!"

Betty Lawson removed 35 pounds of fat, maintained for 5 years, and is a breast cancer survivor

"My Peeke Week Retreat adventure hike to the summit of Aspen's Green Mountain . . . allowed me to seize the opportunity for a few days to leave chemotherapy behind, to breathe in every moment with love, to find the greatest imaginable joy in the beauty of nature. . . . I remember reaching the summit of the mountain and gazing at the unspeakable beauty of the vast panorama of mountaintops that surrounded me, amazed at my accomplishment. It was then that I suddenly realized that any worried thoughts about cancer were gone. Instead, I was filled with a peaceful calm as I became aware of the power of my body and the strength of my mind. I can do anything."

3. Clean It Up!

Flex your environmental muscles and start making some changes to detoxify and optimize your environment. What that means depends not only on your living situation, but also on your financial one. Tired of living in a cement world? Consider moving to one of those wonderful planned wellness communities that are cropping up with running trails or bike paths out the backyard or green spaces to roam. If that's not possible, what can you do to get greater access to nature? Plan weekend trips? Find a park close by? How about planting a garden, even a community garden, and celebrating every seedling's success?

What about the indoors? How can you take those deep cleansing breaths of the Fit to Live lifestyle when you're inhaling toxins and chemicals that make you gag? Do you smoke? Come on, give it up, for heaven's sake! Get help. Try the nicotine replacements— patches or gum—to help with cravings. There are now medications available through your doctor to help wean you off this terribly health-destructive habit. If you're not a smoker, but you're being exposed to secondhand smoke in your environment, stand up for yourself. Ask the person to either put the cigarette out or go somewhere else.

Detoxifying may mean staying away from as many chemical cleaners, air fresheners, etc., as you can. Declog your drains with boiling water. Wash windows with 2 teaspoons of vinegar to 1 quart of water. Eliminate pesticides—you can get rid of most bugs on household plants, for instance, by spraying them with a mixture of half water and half detergent. Buy the unscented laundry detergent the next time yours runs out. Buy bottled water instead of drinking tap, or get a water filter for your kitchen faucet.

None of us will completely eliminate all toxic exposures or create the ideal living and working situation. Just do the best you can. For more ideas and resources, go to the Macrocosm section in www.drpeeke.com.

4. Travel with Your Portable Fit to Live Environment

People are constantly traveling, whether for work or for pleasure. That means a disruption in your home life and potentially a feeling of loss of control over your environment. A hotel, no matter how nice, is not home. For all you road warriors out there, my advice is to take some of your Fit to Live environment right along with you to keep you mentally in touch as well as more calm and peaceful when you are reminded of the love and support waiting for you at home.

Fascinating FAToid

Nature Helps Remove Mental Fat

Being out in nature, even in a small garden or looking at a tree, has been shown to relieve mental fatigue and create a more positive mood. It's the number one preferred location to de-stress. **Bottom line:** Go for the nature calm rather than the candy calm. It's better for Mind and Mouth!

For example, I bring a little alarm clock with a picture of my hubby, Mark, attached to it. It helps me feel good when I'm lonely for home. I also love to bring my fitness tubing. It weighs almost nothing and allows me to stretch anywhere. I also bring aromatherapy, usually in the form of a small mist spray that I can use in my room. I also have a lavender-scented eye pillow, my journal, and my MP3 player with soothing music. That way, I create a whole environment for myself. You can too.

5. You've Got to Stick Up for Yourself

A congressional assistant once came to see me. She worked in a small, windowless office with the usual in-your-face government fluorescent lighting. Her toxic work environment was killing her. I was helping her think about better self-care—she wasn't eating right or exercising and had the Toxic Belly Fat along with increased blood pressure to prove it. Here was the problem. Everyone in her office came in before dawn and left way after dark. She was absolutely terrified about leaving at 6 p.m. instead of 9. I said, "Just try it once. Get all

Fascinating FAToid

Nature Can Help Trim That Waistline

Check this out: A professor who led wilderness retreats did a study of the effects. Here's what he found: Ninety percent said it helped them break an addiction to food or nicotine! In addition, 90 percent of those who went felt a greater sense of aliveness, energy, and well-being, 77 percent had a major life change upon returning (in relationships, housing, employment, or lifestyle), and 38 percent of those changes were still in effect 5 years later! **Bottom line:** Research now supports the healing power of nature.

your work done, then get up and leave at 6." Well, she got some glares from other people who were work addicted, but she did it. She took a walk. She ate dinner on time. She got some great sleep. She felt so good that she began to do it on a routine basis. Since her productivity was excellent, there was nothing for anyone to complain about. One of her peers did rag on her, but she confronted him head on, fighting for her right to self-care.

> "That's the thing about Mother Nature, she really doesn't care what economic bracket you're in."
> —*Whoopi Goldberg*

What about you? There may be all kinds of things in your environment that work against your taking good care of yourself. It might be where you live. Or your work hours. Or a nagging sister-in-law or coworker. But like this congressional assistant, *you* are in charge of your life. You have the right to make the choices that are best for you. Don't allow your environment—people, places, or things—to stand in your way of your commitment to becoming Fit to Live.

⇒Fit to Live Essentials⇐

Using your score from the "Are You Environmentally Fit to Live?" test, you'll continue to build your individual program with the tips below. As in previous chapters, you'll begin according to your current level.

TO SURVIVE:

If you received a score of 0 to 6 on the test, focus your energy here first. Once you've mastered these, feel free to move up to the tips in "To Enjoy."

1. Walk a Dog Twice a Day, Even if You Don't Have One

That's a line I learned from cardiologist Paul Dudley White. I LOVE it! I cannot begin to tell you how many of my patients have lived in their neighborhoods for 10 years and have no idea of what they're like. Slap on the sunscreen and get out there on your two legs. If it's not safe, or if you want more variety, explore the natural places around your city or town. No matter where you live, there is a park somewhere nearby. My South Central LA family, the Holmeses, found one about 2 miles from home where they walk their dog and throw a ball. Bike, walk, take your Frisbees with you, take the dog, take the kids and the strollers. Don't know where a park is? Go to www.active.com—put in the ZIP code, and it will give you nearby parks.

2. Detox the Losers from Your Life

Your environment is not just a bunch of inanimate objects. It also involves people. Are there people in your life who do nothing but throw up roadblocks in your ability to be Fit to Live? Time to rid your life of the people who are standing in your way. Realistically, it's not like you can just blow everyone off. You're stuck with some—in-laws, bosses, family members. I'm simply saying limit the time you're with them and don't get sucked into their destructive dramas. It costs too many Body Dollars in self-destructive habits and eventually more Toxic Belly Fat. Say to yourself, "Being with toxic people doesn't work for me." We're back to that choice issue again. Say to yourself, "I choose to be with people who support my quest to become Fit to Live." Then fearlessly take the steps necessary to get all the love and nurturing you can.

3. Conserve Those Natural Body Dollars

Nature plays a key role as a green bank of Body Dollar reserves. Every time you get out and soothe your mind while invigorating your body, you're gifting yourself with green Body Dollars. Bank 'em for any crisis in your life. While you sit in a hospital bed with chemotherapy dripping into your veins, tap into your reserves and remember the quiet and beauty of that stream you hiked along, or that breathtaking beach sunset, or that panorama from the summit of a mountain. Doing this modulates your stress hormones and allows your immune system to function more optimally under this medical stress. Being in nature and treasuring the memories are both deeply healing when your mind, body, and spirit need healing the most.

4. Plant Something Green

It could be indoors or outdoors. Or both. It's a wonderful way not only to get closer to nature, but also to teach yourself patience. Ah, patience. When you start to think you can drop your Toxic Belly Fat overnight, plant a seed. You'll see nature at work, and this is the same nature

Fascinating FATroid

Walking Fido Is Good for Your Waist

Guess what researchers found when they gave people dogs and told them to work up to walking them for 20 minutes 5 days a week for a year? An average weight removal of 14 pounds, without changing diet at all! **Bottom line:** Dog or no, get out there!

that controls you. Growth is a slow, magnificent process. It's not something you can rush. I planted 200 Wye oaks on my farm and watched the seedlings become 30-foot trees. I've never felt prouder. It has given me a great sense of accomplishment, as well as humbled me. I've learned the patience it takes to grow, whether you're an oak or a human being.

> "Nature has a great simplicity and therefore a great beauty."
> —*Richard Feynman*

TO ENJOY:

If you scored a 7 to 13 on the test, just take a quick look at the "To Survive" suggestions. If you feel you have them covered, you can start here.

1. Retreat into Nature

I started my Peeke Week Retreats in 2001. Since that time, I have helped guide many nature-deficient souls as they take their first steps into a natural setting. I remember with a smile on my face as I hiked with one group at Red Mountain in St. George, Utah. As we were about to reach the summit of the mountain, one of my hikers, a 53-year-old school principal who had full Toxic Belly Fat Syndrome (diabetes, heart disease) and had never hiked in nature, suddenly stopped and looked concerned. I ran to her, and she quietly noted that she had to go to the bathroom. I pointed to the bushes. She appeared panicked. Handing her some toilet paper, I gently pushed her in the right direction. A few minutes later, she emerged from behind the bushes with a gleeful smile and, as loud as she could, shouted, "I pee'd in the bushes!"

For the rest of the trip, she was more open, more fearless. When she returned from her trip, she kept pictures of herself at the mountain summit on her desk reminding her of that transformative toileting. She stopped dissociating and began to pay attention to her self-care. Plan your own retreat today. Pitch a tent in your own backyard to start. But don't stop there—scope out an organized nature adventure, whether it's a yoga retreat or a backpacking adventure into the wilderness. Go to www.drpeeke.com under Macrocosm to find out how to join me on my next Peeke Week Retreat. Embrace the joy of being outside.

2. Play with Nature

Have you ever kayaked? What about rock climbing? Any hiking, walking, biking, or rowing clubs out there? If not, how about forming your own? What about ecotourism?

Wouldn't it be great to experience nature while learning about the ecology of that environment? If you really want to enjoy nature and play with all that she has to offer, log onto www.sierraclub.org, http://gorp.away.com/index.html, or www.classicjourneys.com.

TO CHALLENGE:

If you scored a 14 to 20 on the test, just take a quick look at the "To Survive" and "To Enjoy" tips. If you feel you have them covered, you can start here.

1. Fight for a Healthy Environment

This isn't a call to arms—and legs for nothing. We need to fight for more bike paths and sidewalks and green space. We need to lobby for building housing developments and offices around public transit stops. Yes, it would cost money, but the rising health-care costs of our being Unfit to Live are threatening state budgets. So the more that communities can become bikeable and walkable, our increased lifestyle fitness will actually save money in the long run, as well as countless Body Dollars in distress, disability, and disease. Call or e-mail your legislators today. Start by logging onto www.epa.gov and choose what topic (recycling, lumbering) interests you most. Then pick up the phone and get active. Or pick up that hammer and join forces with groups like Habitat for Humanity and take an active role in building safe and environmentally healthy homes. Log onto www.habitat.org to learn more. Or cut down that dead tree in your neighborhood and plant another. Get a community garden going. When you give to the environment, you not only get the Body Dollars from increased strength and endurance, but also the gift of peace and connection with nature.

2. Teach Your Children

Remember the Crosby, Stills, Nash, and Young song "Teach Your Children"? The greatest gifts you can ever give those precious kids in your life are your love and your guidance to a healthy lifestyle. Kids care if you're walking the talk. If you're at the Fit to Live to Challenge level, you're not only walkin' it, you're running with it. Take your children along with you when you volunteer to work in community gardens or go to public meetings about trail planning. Reward them with adventures into our magnificent national parks. Fight for more outdoor physical activity in schools. You'll feel the exhilarating joy of knowing that each child is Fit to Live a full and healthy life.

AFTERWORD
THERE IS NO FINISH LINE

Congratulations on completing the book. You're locked and loaded with the basic knowledge you'll need to live well. Now when I ask, are you Fit to Live . . . *to Survive, to Enjoy, to Challenge?* no matter what shape you were in when you opened this book, you can now shout, "You better believe it!" You've cut Mental Fat, Toxic Belly Fat, Financial Fat, and Environmental Fat from a Toxic Lifestyle. You're in better shape to save your own life if you had to and have reduced not only your waistline but your odds of disability and disease. You understand the secret of A^2-ing it every day of your life. You're banking Body Dollar reserves to live long and well. You get it that only those who can adapt to life's ever-changing environment will survive, live independently, and rejoice in their ability to stay Alert and Vertical.

There is no finish line in the Fit to Live life. Use this book as your ongoing companion and guide to help you regroup and refocus when life's stresses challenge you and throw you way out of your comfort zone. Go back and retake the tests at the beginning of each section to see just how far you've come. Then challenge yourself in the areas where you still need work. And be sure to visit me at my Web site (www.drpeeke.com) for ongoing support and updated information as you continue your Fit to Live journey.

From this moment on, wake up in the morning and say, "I take myself on!" Then, armed with love and patience, keep reminding yourself, "If not now, *when*?" Then jump into your life and make it your mission to become leaner, stronger, and more fearless—to become Fit to Live for *life!*

CHARTS FOR MUSCLE TESTS

CARDIORESPIRATORY FITNESS RATING

The following two tests are screening tools that provide an estimate of cardiorespiratory fitness for a 1-mile walk and a 1.5-mile run. They are not as accurate as tests that include an electronic heart rate monitor. They are fine for the purposes of home testing for cardio fitness. Use this chart to help you complete question 2 in the endurance test on page 138.

1-Mile Walk				
RATING	MINUTES (BY GENDER AND AGE)			
	Men Under 40	**Men Over 40**	**Women Under 40**	**Women Over 40**
Excellent	13:00 or less	14:00 or less	13:30 or less	14:30 or less
Good	13:01–15:30	14:01–16:30	13:31–16:00	14:31–17:00
Average	15:31–18:00	16:31–19:00	16:01–18:30	17:01–19:30
Below average	18:01–19:30	19:01–21:30	18:31–20:00	19:31–22:00
Low	19:31 or more	21:31 or more	20:01 or more	22:01 or more

Date:_____

Your Fit to Live Cardiorespiratory Rating (circle one):

EXCELLENT   GOOD   AVERAGE   BELOW AVERAGE   LOW

Reference: *Walking Handbook*, Susan Johnson, EdD; The Cooper Institute, 2000.

Use one of the following two charts to help you complete question 3 in the endurance test on page 138.

Female 1.5-Mile Run						
TIME (BY AGE GROUP IN MINUTES)						RATING
Ages 20–29	Ages 30–39	Ages 40–49	Ages 50–59	Ages 60–69	Ages 70–79	
9:23	9:52	10:09	11:34	12:25	12:25	**Superior**
10:20	11:08	11:35	13:16	14:28	14:33	
10:59	11:43	12:25	13:58	15:32	16:06	**Excellent**
11:34	12:23	13:14	14:33	16:22	16:57	
11:56	12:53	13:38	15:14	16:46	18:05	
12:07	13:08	13:58	15:47	17:34	18:39	**Good**
12:51	13:41	14:33	16:26	18:05	19:24	
13:01	13:58	15:03	16:46	18:39	20:02	
13:25	14:33	15:17	17:19	18:52	20:54	
13:58	14:33	15:56	17:38	19:29	21:45	**Fair**
14:15	15:14	16:13	18:05	20:08	22:22	
14:33	15:35	16:46	18:39	20:38	22:54	
15:05	15:56	17:11	19:10	20:55	23:47	
15:32	16:43	17:38	19:43	22:03	24:54	**Poor**
15:56	16:46	18:26	20:17	22:34	25:49	
16:43	17:38	18:39	20:55	23:20	26:15	
17:11	18:18	19:43	21:57	23:55	27:17	
17:53	19:01	20:49	22:53	25:02	27:55	**Very poor**
18:39	20:13	21:52	23:55	26:32	30:34	
21:05	21:57	23:27	26:15	29:06	33:32	
25:17	25:10	27:55	30:34	33:05	37:26	

Male 1.5-Mile Run						
TIME (BY AGE GROUP IN MINUTES)						RATING
Ages 20–29	Ages 30–39	Ages 40–49	Ages 50–59	Ages 60–69	Ages 70–79	
8:22	8:49	9:02	9:31	10:09	10:27	**Superior**
9:10	9:31	9:47	10:27	11:20	12:25	
9:34	9:52	10:09	11:09	12:10	13:25	**Excellent**
9:52	10:14	10:44	11:45	12:53	13:57	
10:08	10:38	11:09	12:08	13:25	14:52	
10:34	10:59	11:32	12:37	13:58	15:38	**Good**
10:49	11:09	11:52	12:53	14:33	16:22	
11:09	11:34	11:58	13:25	14:55	16:46	
11:27	11:49	12:25	13:53	15:20	17:37	
11:34	11:58	12:53	13:58	15:53	18:05	**Fair**
11:58	12:25	13:05	14:33	16:19	18:39	
12:11	12:44	13:25	14:35	16:46	19:19	
12:29	12:53	13:50	15:14	17:19	19:43	
12:53	13:25	14:10	15:53	17:49	20:28	**Poor**
13:08	13:48	14:33	16:16	18:39	21:28	
13:25	14:10	15:00	16:46	19:10	22:22	
13:58	14:33	15:32	17:30	20:13	23:55	
14:33	15:14	16:09	18:22	21:34	25:49	**Very poor**
15:14	15:56	17:04	19:24	23:27	27:55	
16:46	17:30	18:39	21:40	25:58	30:34	
20:55	20:55	22:22	27:08	31:59	33:30	

DYNAMIC STRENGTH TEST

This test is a screening tool that provides an estimate of your dynamic strength. Use this chart to help you complete question 3 in the strength test on page 140.

	MALES					FEMALES					RATING
PERCENTAGE	NUMBER OF PUSHUPS (BY AGE GROUP)					NUMBER OF MODIFIED PUSHUPS (BY AGE GROUP)					
	Ages 20–29	Ages 30–39	Ages 40–49	Ages 50–59	Age 60+	Ages 20–29	Ages 30–39	Ages 40–49	Ages 50–59	Age 60+	
99	100	86	64	51	39	70	56	60	31	20	**Superior**
95	62	52	40	39	28	45	39	33	28	20	
90	57	46	36	30	26	42	36	28	25	17	**Excellent**
85	51	41	34	28	24	39	33	26	23	15	
80	47	39	30	25	23	36	31	24	21	15	
75	44	36	29	24	22	34	29	21	20	15	**Good**
70	41	34	26	21	21	32	28	20	19	14	
65	39	31	25	20	20	31	26	19	18	13	
60	37	30	24	19	18	30	24	18	17	12	
55	35	29	22	17	16	29	23	17	15	12	**Fair**
50	33	27	21	15	15	26	21	15	13	8	
45	31	25	19	14	12	25	20	14	13	6	
40	29	24	18	13	10	23	19	13	12	5	
35	27	21	16	11	9	22	17	11	10	4	**Poor**
30	26	20	15	10	8	20	15	10	9	3	
25	24	19	13	9.5	7	19	14	9	8	2	
20	22	17	11	9	6	17	11	6	6	2	
15	19	15	10	7	5	15	9	4	4	1	**Very Poor**
10	18	13	9	6	4	12	8	2	1	0	
5	13	9	5	3	2	9	4	1	0	0	

THE FIT TO LIVE TRACKING FORMS

These handy forms will help you become Fit to Live. The first chart, the Body Composition Tracker, allows you to watch the pounds and inches come off as your body composition improves. Make a copy of this form or just note the changes right here in your book. The second chart, the Fit to Live template, organizes your Fit to Live plan every day. Make 28 copies of this chart for your first 4 weeks and copy more thereafter, as needed. Every day, note the Fit to Live Principles and Essentials you'll focus on that day. Use the Mouth and Muscle sections to keep track of your eating and exercise. Don't forget: research shows people who journal are more successful in their weight removal efforts!

BASELINE STATS	WEEK 1 __/__/__	WEEK 2 __/__/__	WEEK 3 __/__/__	WEEK 4 __/__/__	WEEK 5 __/__/__	WEEK 6 __/__/__
Weight:						
Body Fat %:						
CURRENT SIZES						
Men (belt size):						
Women (jeans size):						
CLOTHES-O-METER*						
Men Size:	☐ too tight ☐ just right	☐ too tight ☐ just right	☐ too tight ☐ just right	☐ too tight ☐ just right	☐ too tight ☐ just right	☐ too tight ☐ just right
Women Size:	☐ too tight ☐ just right	☐ too tight ☐ just right	☐ too tight ☐ just right	☐ too tight ☐ just right	☐ too tight ☐ just right	☐ too tight ☐ just right
MEASUREMENTS (circumference in inches)						
Waist (across belly button):						
Hip-Buttock:						
Chest (women, below breasts):						
Thighs (mid-thigh): Left / Right						
Upper Arms (mid-arm): Left / Right						

* An article of clothing that you can put on but is too tight to wear in public and that you will use to monitor your progress each week.

DATE ___/___/___	TODAY'S FIT TO LIVE **PRINCIPLES**	TODAY'S FIT TO LIVE **ESSENTIALS**
MIND	Cut Mental Fat	
	Practice Safe Stress	
MOUTH	Focus on Quality	
	Rein in Quantity	
	Increase Frequency	
	Stop Dieting	
MUSCLE	Move toward Endurance	
	Push for Strength	
	Reach for Flexibility and Balance	
MONEY	Make Body/Bank Dollar Connection	
	Refire and Rejoice	
MACROCOSM	Conquer Clutter	
	Get Outside	

MENUS WITH RECIPES FOR MEAT EATERS

Day 1

Breakfast

Top ¾ cup **Back to Nature Hi-Fiber Multibran Cereal** with ½ **sliced banana** and ½ **cup low-fat (1%) milk**. Serve with **a hard-cooked egg**.

Breakfast total: 323 calories, 16 g protein, 60 g carbohydrate, 8 g fat, 3 g saturated fat, 217 mg cholesterol, 215 mg sodium, 13 g dietary fiber.

Morning Snack

A **6-oz low-fat drinkable yogurt** (such as Dannon or Yoplait)

Snack total: 153 calories, 7 g protein, 27 g carbohydrate, 3 g fat, 2 g saturated fat, 9 mg cholesterol, 94 mg sodium, 0 g dietary fiber.

Lunch

Quick Tortilla (serves 1): Drizzle **1 high-protein tortilla** (such as La Tortilla Factory) **with olive oil**, and top with **1 whole roasted pepper**, ⅓ **cup grated low-fat mozzarella or feta cheese**, and **a sprinkling of dried herb mix** such as Mrs. Dash. Top brown for 5 minutes.

Lunch total: 361 calories, 19 g protein, 59 g carbohydrate, 12 g fat, 5 g saturated fat, 20 mg cholesterol, 627 mg sodium, 7 g dietary fiber.

Afternoon Snack

Serve **1 medium toasted whole wheat pita** with 1 serving **(2 Tbsp) Black Bean Hummus** (see recipe below)

Black Bean Hummus (serves 6): Mix in a blender or food processor **one 15-oz can black beans**, drained, **3 Tbsp lemon juice, 1 tsp crushed garlic, 3 Tbsp tahini**, and **1 Tbsp olive oil**. Garnish with **2 Tbsp parsley** and a drizzle of additional **olive oil**.

Snack total per person: 250 calories, 10 g protein, 37 g carbohydrate, 8 g fat, 1 g saturated fat, 0 mg cholesterol, 466 mg sodium, 8 g dietary fiber.

Dinner

Mixed Seafood Salad (serves 1): Combine ¼ lb thawed, **frozen cooked seafood mix**, such as lobster, shrimp, scallops, and squid, with **1 cup romaine lettuce or spinach, ½ cup artichoke hearts, some finely chopped raw broccoli, cucumber, red peppers, and scallions, ½ medium orange**, segmented, and **a few black olives**. Add **Mrs. Dash seasoning, scant olive oil**, and **fresh lemon juice**. Toss and serve.

Dinner total: 360 calories, 29 g protein, 35 g carbohydrate, 13 g fat, 2 g saturated fat, 101 mg cholesterol, 619 mg sodium, 13 g dietary fiber.

Day 1 total: *1,447 calories, 81 g protein, 218 g carbohydrate, 44 g fat, 13 g saturated fat, 347 mg cholesterol, 2,021 mg sodium, 41 g dietary fiber.*

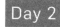

Day 2

Breakfast

Egg Beaters Omelet with Cheese (serves 1): Cook **1 cup Egg Beaters** in a nonstick pan for about 7 minutes or until set in center. Top with ⅓ **cup grated fat-free cheese**, and fold omelet in half. Serve with a **2-cup mix of fresh melon**, such as cantaloupe, honeydew, and watermelon.

Breakfast total: 280 calories, 38 g protein, 31 g carbohydrate, 1 g fat, 0 g saturated fat, 7 mg cholesterol, 786 mg sodium, 2 g dietary fiber.

Morning Snack

A banana and **3 or 4 walnuts**

Snack total: 152 calories, 2 g protein, 28 g carbohydrate, 5 g fat, 1 g saturated fat, 0 mg cholesterol, 2 mg sodium, 3 g dietary fiber.

⬊ *Lunch*

Prepare a sandwich with **2 slices whole grain bread**, **3 slices Oscar Mayer fat-free lunch meat**, **a slice of fat-free cheese** (American or Swiss), **mustard**, **lettuce**, and **alfalfa sprouts**. Serve with **about 10 baked chips or soy crisps**. (To reduce sodium, choose low-sodium lunch meat, cheese, and chips.)

Lunch total: 376 calories, 30 g protein, 54 g carbohydrate, 6 g fat, 1 g saturated fat, 27 mg cholesterol, 1,858 mg sodium, 7 g dietary fiber.

⬊ *Afternoon Snack*

About 10 whole wheat pretzels and a ¼-cup mix of raisins and peanuts.

Snack total: 270 calories, 7 g protein, 54 g carbohydrate, 6 g fat, 1 g saturated fat, 0 mg cholesterol, 143 mg sodium, 4 g dietary fiber.

⬊ *Dinner*

Grilled Salmon with Chili Seasoning (serves 4): Stir together in a small bowl **¼ cup ground paprika, 1 Tbsp chili powder, 1 Tbsp ground cumin, 1 tsp salt, ¼ tsp cinnamon, and ¼ tsp ground red pepper**. Pat 2 Tbsp of this spice mix over the flesh side of a **1½-lb salmon fillet**. Place fish in a fish basket and grill over medium heat for about 6 minutes. Turn over and grill for 5 to 6 minutes longer. Remove and cut into four portions. Serve with **lemon wedges**.

> **Fresh Tomato and Cucumber Salad (serves 4)**: Chop **2 medium cucumbers** and **4 medium tomatoes** and mix with **parsley, cilantro, vinegar,** and **salt** to taste.

> **Green Beans with Sautéed Mushrooms (serves 4)**: Steam 1 lb trimmed **green beans** until crisp-cooked. Sauté **½ lb mushrooms** in **1 tsp olive oil** for 5 minutes. Stir in green beans and add **garlic powder, salt,** and **pepper**.

Dinner total per person: 484 calories, 53 g protein, 21 g carbohydrate, 22 g fat, 4 g saturated fat, 148 mg cholesterol, 738 mg sodium, 8 g dietary fiber.

....

Day 2 total: *1,562 calories, 130 g protein, 188 g carbohydrate, 40 g fat, 7 g saturated fat, 182 mg cholesterol, 3,527 mg sodium, 24 g dietary fiber.*

Day 3

⬎ *Breakfast*

Yogurt French Toast (serves 2): Beat **1 whole egg** with **2 egg whites, ½ cup fat-free milk,** and **¼ tsp cinnamon**. Soak **4 slices whole grain bread** in egg mixture for 2 minutes. Cook over medium heat in a nonstick skillet, lightly coated with **olive oil**, and turn slices. Top with mix of **1 cup fat-free yogurt, 2 Tbsp maple syrup**, and **1 cup coarsely chopped fresh fruit,** such as strawberries, kiwifruits, bananas, and peaches.

Breakfast total per person: 404 calories, 22 g protein, 65 g carbohydrate, 8 g fat, 2 g saturated fat, 110 mg cholesterol, 540 mg sodium, 6 g dietary fiber.

⬎ *Morning Snack*

An apple with **1 Tbsp almond butter.**

Snack total: 183 calories, 3 g protein, 24 g carbohydrate, 10 g fat, 1 g saturated fat, 0 mg cholesterol, 2 mg sodium, 4 g dietary fiber.

⬎ *Lunch*

Canned Tuna and Chickpea Salad with Gazpacho (serves 4): Combine **one 6-oz can tuna** with **one 15-oz can chickpeas,** drained. Add **½ cup chopped scallions, ¼ cup chopped parsley,** and **2 tsp balsamic vinegar**. Set aside. Finely chop **2 pickling cucumbers, ½ red onion,** and **1 red pepper**. Mix with **2 cups chopped fresh tomatoes, 1 cup tomato juice,** and **1 Tbsp minced garlic**. Chill the soup 2 hours or overnight. Serve tuna and chickpea salad with **5 or 6 whole grain crackers per person** and chilled soup.

Lunch total per person: 324 calories, 22 g protein, 48 g carbohydrate, 6 g fat, 1 g saturated fat, 13 mg cholesterol, 320 mg sodium, 11 g dietary fiber.

⬎ *Afternoon Snack*

A 6-oz low-fat fruit yogurt and **about 10 soy crisps.**

Snack total: 275 calories, 15 g protein, 47 g carbohydrate, 4 g fat, 1 g saturated fat, 7 mg cholesterol, 362 mg sodium, 2 g dietary fiber.

⤷ *Dinner*

Pork Roast with Spicy Glaze (serves 4): Preheat oven to 350°F. For glaze, whisk together **¼ cup maple syrup, ¼ cup Splenda, 2 Tbsp cider vinegar, 1 Tbsp light soy sauce, salt** and **pepper** to taste. Place a **1-lb boneless pork roast** in a roasting pan and insert a meat thermometer. Coat with glaze. Surround roast with **4 cups vegetables** such as potatoes, carrots, parsnips, winter squash, and onions. Bake until meat thermometer reaches 160°F, about 1 to 1¼ hours.

Dinner total per person: 385 calories, 37 g protein, 37 g carbohydrate, 10 g fat, 4 g saturated fat, 93 mg cholesterol, 407 mg sodium, 5 g dietary fiber.

Day 3 total: *1,571 calories, 99 g protein, 221 g carbohydrate, 38 g fat, 9 g saturated fat, 223 mg cholesterol, 1,631 mg sodium, 28 g dietary fiber.*

Day 4

⤷ *Breakfast*

Turkey Sausage and Vegetable Brunch Casserole (serves 4): Brown **4 oz light turkey sausage** (or soy equivalent to make it vegetarian), separated into small pieces, in a nonstick pan. Turn off heat and add **1½ cups broccoli and 1½ cups red bell pepper,** cut into bite-size pieces, **¼ cup chopped scallions**, and **1 cup shredded Cabot 75% reduced-fat Cheddar cheese**. Spoon mixture into an 8" × 8" baking pan. Beat together **2 eggs, ½ cup egg substitute, ½ cup fat-free ricotta cheese, ¼ tsp Mrs. Dash salt-free seasoning**, and **pepper**. Pour mixture over sausage and vegetables in pan. Thinly slice **1 large tomato** and arrange on top. Cover with foil and bake for 45 minutes at 350°F. Uncover, sprinkle **¼ cup Parmesan cheese** on top and bake 15 minutes longer, uncovered.

Breakfast total per person: 281 calories, 29 g protein, 10 g carbohydrate, 15 g fat, 7 g saturated fat, 155 mg cholesterol, 401 mg sodium, 3 g dietary fiber.

⤷ *Morning Snack*

1½ cups unsweetened applesauce.

Snack total: 157 calories, 1 g protein, 41 g carbohydrate, 0 g fat, 0 g saturated fat, 0 mg cholesterol, 7 mg sodium, 4 g dietary fiber.

⬎ *Lunch*

Quick Tuna Salad (serves 2): Purchase **2 cooked and seasoned 4-oz tuna steaks**. In a large bowl, toss **4 cups shredded romaine lettuce, 1 package grape tomatoes, 1 pickling cucumber,** thinly sliced, and **1 large, sliced roasted pepper from a jar**. In a small bowl, whisk together **juice from ½ lemon, 2 Tbsp olive oil, 1 Tbsp spicy mustard,** and **a few shakes garlic powder**. Arrange the salad onto two plates. Cut the tuna into ½" strips and place on top. Pour dressing over the tuna and sprinkle with **fresh dill.**

Lunch total per person: 384 calories, 32 g protein, 19 g carbohydrate, 21 g fat, 4 g saturated fat, 43 mg cholesterol, 257 mg sodium, 6 g dietary fiber.

⬎ *Afternoon Snack*

A large banana and **¼ cup raisins.**

Snack total: 272 calories, 3 g protein, 70 g carbohydrate, 1 g fat, 0 g saturated fat, 0 mg cholesterol, 6 mg sodium, 6 g dietary fiber.

⬎ *Dinner*

Pepper Steak in 10 Minutes (serves 2): Microwave **¼ cup Uncle Ben's Quick Brown Rice,** following package directions. Place into a sturdy freezer-style bag **½ lb sirloin steak,** cut into strips, **1 cup green bell pepper,** cut into 1" pieces, **1 large Vidalia onion,** cut into 1" pieces, **1 small package frozen sugar snap peas, 2 Tbsp low-sodium soy sauce, 2 tsp olive oil, ½ tsp garlic powder,** and **1 tsp red pepper flakes** or **½ tsp ground red pepper**. Close bag and shake vigorously until meat and vegetables are well coated. Pour into hot skillet and stir-fry 3 to 4 minutes. Serve over rice.

Dinner total per person: 488 calories, 43 g protein, 45 g carbohydrate, 15 g fat, 4 g saturated fat, 101 mg cholesterol, 630 mg sodium, 9 g dietary fiber.

....

Day 4 total: *1,582 calories, 108 g protein, 185 g carbohydrate, 52 g fat, 15 g saturated fat, 299 mg cholesterol, 1,301 mg sodium, 28 g dietary fiber.*

Day 5

Breakfast

Serve ½ **cup cooked Kashi Breakfast Pilaf** with **1 scrambled egg or egg substitute** and **4 oz calcium-fortified orange juice**.

Breakfast total: 300 calories, 13 g protein, 44 g carbohydrate, 8 g fat, 2 g saturated fat, 213 mg cholesterol, 78 mg sodium, 6 g dietary fiber.

Morning Snack

A large pear and **1 oz low-fat Cheddar cheese**.

Snack total: 176 calories, 8 g protein, 33 g carbohydrate, 3 g fat, 1 g saturated fat, 6 mg cholesterol, 6 mg sodium, 5 g dietary fiber.

Lunch

Soup and ½ Sandwich (serves 1): Prepare **½ can minestrone soup** such as Progresso. On **2 slices whole grain bread,** place **4 thin slices smoked turkey, 2 slices light Swiss cheese, ½ sliced tomato,** and **½ cup baby spinach** or **broccoli sprouts.** If desired, add **2 tsp Spectrum organic mayonnaise with omega-3 fat.** Cut sandwich in half to enjoy for 2 days.

Lunch total (with mayonnaise): 355 calories, 24 g protein, 43 g carbohydrate, 11 g fat, 3 g saturated fat, 38 mg cholesterol, 1,359 mg sodium, 4 g dietary fiber.

Afternoon Snack

6 or 7 Wasa crackers with **1 Tbsp peanut butter.**

Snack total: 262 calories, 9 g protein, 34 g carbohydrate, 11 g fat, 2 g saturated fat, 0 mg cholesterol, 342 mg sodium, 4 g dietary fiber.

Dinner

Curried Chicken Kabobs with Coconut Rice, prepared ahead of time **(serves 4)**: Cut **1 lb chicken tenders** into large chunks and mix in a bowl with **1 cup fat-free plain yogurt, ½ cup light coconut milk, 1 Tbsp curry powder, 1 tsp crushed**

garlic, **2 tsp fresh lemon juice**, and if desired, **salt** and **pepper**. Refrigerate for several hours. Preheat broiler or grill. Cut **2 large Spanish onions** into chunks. Alternate chicken on skewers with onions. Prepare **1½ cups cooked basmati** or **jasmine brown rice** according to package directions, substituting **1 cup coconut milk** for 1 cup water. Add **½ cup green peas**, fresh or frozen, during the last 5 minutes of cooking. Grill or broil kabobs until cooked through, and serve over rice.

Dinner total per person: 339 calories, 34 g protein, 31 g carbohydrate, 9 g fat, 6 g saturated fat, 67 mg cholesterol, 156 mg sodium, 4 g dietary fiber.

Day 5 total: *1,432 calories, 88 g protein, 185 g carbohydrate, 42 g fat, 14 g saturated fat, 324 mg cholesterol, 1,941 mg sodium, 23 g dietary fiber.*

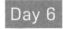
Day 6

⬧ *Breakfast*

Serve **1 high-protein Bran Muffin** (see recipe below) with **1 hard-cooked egg** and **10 oz low-sugar cranberry juice**.

> **Bran Muffins (makes 24):** The batter may be made ahead and refrigerated. Combine **1½ cups wheat bran** and **1 cup boiling water**. Blend **1¼ cups whole wheat flour**, **½ cup soy flour**, **½ cup all-purpose flour**, **2 Tbsp flax meal**, **2½ tsp baking soda**, and **½ tsp salt**. Wisk into bran mixture **⅓ cup honey**, **⅓ cup molasses**, **½ cup Splenda**, **¼ cup canola**, **flax**, or **olive oil** and **2 large eggs**, beaten (or **¼ cup Egg Beaters**). Stir in **1⅓ cups chopped dried fruit** (such as raisins, blueberries, figs, prunes, or apricots) and **1 cup coarsely chopped walnuts**. Add the flour mixture and blend until barely moistened. Fill greased or paper-lined muffin tins. Bake at 400°F for about 16 minutes or until a toothpick inserted into the center comes out clean. Wrap tightly after cooling to keep muffins from drying out.

Breakfast total per person: 292 calories, 10 g protein, 37 g carbohydrate, 12 g fat, 3 g saturated fat, 230 mg cholesterol, 259 mg sodium, 4 g dietary fiber.

Morning Snack

A 6-oz low-fat mixed berry yogurt.

Snack total: 173 calories, 7 g protein, 32 g carbohydrate, 2 g fat, 1 g saturated fat, 11 mg cholesterol, 94 mg sodium, 0 g dietary fiber.

Lunch

Spicy Shrimp (serves 4): Combine **1 lb cooked medium shrimp** with **juice from 3 limes** and **1 cup salsa**. Chill for at least 30 minutes, then add **1 chopped pickling cucumber, ¼ cup finely chopped celery, 1 ripe chopped avocado**, and **1 small hot pepper,** thinly sliced. Line a serving bowl with **2 cups fresh spinach and/or Bibb lettuce leaves**. Place shrimp mix on the lettuce. Serve with **1 oz low-fat tortilla chips** per person, if desired.

Lunch total per person (with chips): 347 calories, 33 g protein, 38 g carbohydrate, 11 g fat, 2 g saturated fat, 221 mg cholesterol, 700 mg sodium, 10 g dietary fiber.

Afternoon Snack

A large apple and **2 sticks low-fat string cheese.**

Snack total: 284 calories, 16 g protein, 34 g carbohydrate, 10 g fat, 6 g saturated fat, 31 mg cholesterol, 299 mg sodium, 6 g dietary fiber.

Dinner

Oven-Fried Chicken (serves 4): Marinate the chicken 4 to 24 hours in advance. Combine **1 lb skinless chicken pieces** and **1 cup low-fat buttermilk** in a gallon-size zip-top bag. Refrigerate for several hours or overnight. When ready to cook, arrange oven racks to accommodate 2 baking sheets and preheat oven to 400°F. Mix **1 cup whole wheat flour, ½ tsp ground chipotle** or **ground red pepper, ¼ tsp ground cumin, salt** and **pepper** in a large bowl, and add chicken, one piece at a time, to coat thoroughly. Holding each chicken piece over a baking sheet, spray both sides with **canola** or **olive oil spray**. Dip into flour mixture a second time and spray again. Place each piece bone side down onto the baking sheet. Bake for about 40 minutes until golden brown.

Oven-Baked Garlic Fries (serves 4): These may be baked at the same time and temperature as the chicken. Preheat oven to 400°F. Coat a baking sheet with **canola cooking spray.** Combine **1½ lb peeled potatoes,** cut into ¼" strips, **2 tsp vegetable oil, ½ tsp garlic powder,** and ¼ tsp seasoned salt in a zip-top bag. Shake to coat. Arrange in a single layer on the baking sheet. Bake for about 40 minutes or until tender and golden brown. Place into a serving dish and top with **1 Tbsp finely chopped parsley** and **2 Tbsp grated Parmesan cheese.**

Homemade Coleslaw (serves 4): Combine **2 cups coarsely grated mix of fresh cabbage, carrot, celery, and bell pepper** with **2 Tbsp vinegar, 1 Tbsp light mayonnaise,** and **2 Tbsp plain yogurt.**

Dinner total per person: 517 calories, 37 g protein, 64 g carbohydrate, 13 g fat, 3 g saturated fat, 72 mg cholesterol, 364 mg sodium, 8 g dietary fiber.

Day 6 total: *1,613 calories, 103 g protein, 205 g carbohydrate, 48 g fat, 15 g saturated fat, 565 mg cholesterol, 1,716 mg sodium, 28 g dietary fiber.*

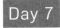

Day 7

⤵ *Breakfast*

Combine **½ cup low-fat cottage or ricotta cheese** with **½ cup unsweetened applesauce.** Top with **½ tsp cinnamon** and **2 Tbsp slivered almonds.**

Breakfast total: 212 calories, 17 g protein, 20 g carbohydrate, 8 g fat, 1 g saturated fat, 5 mg cholesterol, 461 mg sodium, 3 g dietary fiber.

⤵ *Morning Snack*

A medium orange and **1 oz soy nuts.**

Snack total: 182 calories, 13 g protein, 24 g carbohydrate, 4 g fat, 1 g saturated fat, 0 mg cholesterol, 150 mg sodium, 8 g dietary fiber.

⤵ *Lunch*

Prepare **½ cup cooked brown rice** according to package directions. Stir rice into **½ can prepared lentil soup.** Serve with **1 slice crusty bread** and **1 slice low-fat cheese.**

Lunch total: 385 calories, 21 g protein, 62 g carbohydrate, 6 g fat, 2 g saturated fat, 6 mg cholesterol, 1,123 mg sodium, 10 g dietary fiber.

⬎ *Afternoon Snack*

Add **a large sliced fresh peach or nectarine** to **1 cup low-fat plain yogurt**. Top with **½ Tbsp wheat germ** and **1 Tbsp crystallized ginger**.

Snack total: 254 calories, 15 g protein, 41 g carbohydrate, 5 g fat, 2 g saturated fat, 14 mg cholesterol, 160 mg sodium, 3 g dietary fiber.

⬎ *Dinner*

Ground Turkey Stew (serves 4): Brown **1 lb ground turkey** and drain off any fat. Add to pan **6 cups mixed vegetables**, fresh or frozen, such as chopped onions, bell peppers, carrots, broccoli, and cauliflower. Add **2 minced garlic cloves**, **¼ tsp cumin**, **salt**, and **pepper to taste**. Continue cooking until vegetables are crisp-cooked.

Dinner total per person: 431 calories, 33 g protein, 53 g carbohydrate, 13 g fat, 3 g saturated fat, 84 mg cholesterol, 257 mg sodium, 13 g dietary fiber.

....

Day 7 total: *1,464 calories, 99 g protein, 200 g carbohydrate, 36 g fat, 9 g saturated fat, 109 mg cholesterol, 2,151 mg sodium, 37 g dietary fiber.*

SHOPPING LIST FOR MENUS FOR MEAT EATERS

- **Seafood**: 8 oz tuna steak, several 6 oz cans tuna, 1½ lb salmon fillet, 1 lb cooked shrimp, ¼ lb frozen seafood mix (such as lobster, shrimp, scallops, and squid).
- **Meat**: 1 lb boneless pork roast, ½ lb sirloin steak, 1 lb ground turkey, 4 oz light turkey sausage, 1 lb skinless chicken, 1 lb chicken tenders, 6 to 8 oz sliced smoked turkey or other lunch meat (such as Oscar Mayer).
- **Dairy products**: ¼ gallon fat-free or low-fat milk, 1 pint low-fat buttermilk, 1 32-oz container fat-free or low-fat plain yogurt, several 6 oz low-fat fruit yogurts and drinkable yogurts, 16 oz low-fat or fat-free cheese, 8 oz low-fat cottage or ½ cup fat-free ricotta cheese, 8 oz Parmesan cheese, low-fat string cheese, 1 cup shredded Cabot 75% reduced-fat Cheddar cheese, ¼ lb light Swiss cheese.

- **Eggs**: 1 dozen eggs, 1 16-oz container Egg Beaters.
- **Vegetables**: 6 to 8 red or green bell peppers, 1 hot pepper, 6 to 8 pickling cucumbers, 1 cauliflower, 1 bunch broccoli, 6 to 8 potatoes, 6 to 8 tomatoes, 1 container grape tomatoes, 1 lb green beans, several large onions and scallions (including Spanish and Vidalia), 1 box mushrooms, 1 head romaine lettuce, 1 container fresh baby spinach, 1 cabbage, several ribs celery, 1 bunch parsley, small container alfalfa or broccoli sprouts, 1 avocado, 1 can artichoke hearts, 2 packages frozen peas, carrots, parsnips, winter squash, 1 jar roasted peppers, 1 package frozen sugar snap peas.
- **Fruit**: Several bananas, oranges, lemons, limes, and apples, 1 fresh cantaloupe, honeydew, or watermelon, several pears, peaches, or kiwifruits, 1 box strawberries, 1 jar unsweetened applesauce, 2 boxes raisins or other dried fruit (such as blueberries, figs, prunes, or apricots).
- **Juice**: Small containers of calcium-fortified orange juice, tomato juice, and low-sugar cranberry juice.
- **Nuts and seeds**: Walnuts, almonds, soy nuts, 1 jar almond butter, 1 jar peanut butter, 1 jar tahini.
- **Legumes**: 1 15-oz can black beans, peanuts, 1 15-oz can chickpeas.
- **Whole grains**: 1 packet whole grain tortillas or pita bread, 1 loaf whole grain bread, 1 box whole grain crackers, small bag whole wheat pretzels, 1 box Uncle Ben's Quick Brown Rice, 1 box Kashi Breakfast Pilaf, 1 box Back to Nature Hi-Fiber Multibran Cereal, 1 loaf crusty bread, tortilla chips, Wasa crackers, 1½ cups jasmine or basmati brown rice.
- **Oils**: Olive oil, canola or olive oil cooking spray.
- **Spices**: Garlic powder, fresh garlic, paprika, chili powder, ground chipotle, cilantro, curry powder, ground cumin, cinnamon, fresh dill, salt, pepper, ground red pepper, crystallized ginger, mustard, a dried herb seasoning such as Mrs. Dash, balsamic or cider vinegar, low-sodium soy sauce, 1 tsp red pepper flakes, seasoned salt.
- **Baking ingredients**: Whole wheat flour, all-purpose flour, soy flour, wheat bran, wheat germ, flax meal, baking soda, maple syrup, honey, molasses, Splenda, 1 pint light coconut milk.
- **Other**: Small container black olives, 1 bag baked chips or soy crisps, 1 container salsa, 1 jar Spectrum organic mayonnaise with omega-3 fat, several cans of prepared soup such as lentil or minestrone.

MENUS WITH RECIPES FOR VEGETARIANS

Day 1

Breakfast

Prepare **1 cup cooked high-protein oatmeal** (such as Quaker Steel Cut Oats) **and top with ¼ cup dried cherries, walnut pieces,** or **fresh blueberries,** and **½ cup kefir or soy milk.**

Breakfast total: 340 calories, 12 g protein, 57 g carbohydrate, 6 g fat, 0 g saturated fat, 0 mg cholesterol, 61 mg sodium, 7 g dietary fiber.

Morning Snack

A hard-cooked egg with **salt** and **pepper** to taste and **1 oz soy crisps.**

Snack total: 179 calories, 13 g protein, 15 g carbohydrate, 7 g fat, 2 g saturated fat, 212 mg cholesterol, 325 mg sodium, 2 g dietary fiber.

Lunch

Tabbouleh (serves 4): Place **1 cup uncooked bulgur** into a small mixing bowl and pour **2 cups boiling water** over it. Mix gently, cover, and allow to sit for 1 hour. Remove excess water by pouring through a strainer and pressing with a wooden spoon. Place drained bulgur in a bowl and mix in **2 medium chopped fresh tomatoes, ¾ cup chopped parsley, 3 Tbsp fresh lemon juice, ⅛ tsp garlic powder, ⅓ cup chopped scallions,** and ¾ **cup drained canned chickpeas.** Cover and refrigerate at least 2 hours before serving with **2 medium slices crusty whole grain bread** per person.

Lunch total per person: 345 calories, 14 g protein, 68 g carbohydrate, 4 g fat, 1 g saturated fat, 0 mg cholesterol, 361 mg sodium, 14 g dietary fiber.

Afternoon Snack

Serve **1 medium toasted whole wheat pita** with 1 serving **Black Bean Hummus** (see recipe below).

Black Bean Hummus (serves 6): Mix in a blender or food processor **1 15-oz can black beans**, drained, **3 Tbsp lemon juice, 1 tsp crushed garlic, 3 Tbsp tahini**, and **1 Tbsp olive oil**. Garnish with **2 Tbsp parsley** and a drizzle of additional **olive oil**.

Snack total per person: 250 calories, 10 g protein, 37 g carbohydrate, 8 g fat, 1 g saturated fat, 0 mg cholesterol, 466 mg sodium, 8 g dietary fiber.

Dinner

Rotini with Vegetables (serves 1): Cook **2 oz rotini pasta** such as Barilla Plus Whole Grain and Legume Blend according to package directions and mix with **1 cup lightly steamed vegetables** such as broccoli, sugar snap peas, and eggplant, and **1 cup roasted vegetables** such as red pepper, acorn squash, red onion, and garlic. Add **1 Tbsp olive oil** and **Mrs. Dash seasoning**, **salt**, and **pepper** to taste.

Dinner total: 491 calories, 15 g protein, 80 g carbohydrate, 16 g fat, 2 g saturated fat, 0 mg cholesterol, 52 mg sodium, 15 g dietary fiber.

....

Day 1 total: *1,605 calories, 64 g protein, 257 g carbohydrate, 41 g fat, 6 g saturated fat, 212 mg cholesterol, 1,265 mg sodium, 46 g dietary fiber.*

Day 2

Breakfast

Prepare **a 3-oz soy sausage patty**. Serve with ½ **small whole grain bagel** topped with **1 tsp light plant sterol spread**, and a glass of ½ **cup pomegranate juice**.

Breakfast total: 341 calories, 21 g protein, 41 g carbohydrate, 11 g fat, 2 g saturated fat, 0 mg cholesterol, 666 mg sodium, 7 g dietary fiber.

Morning Snack

An apple with **1 Tbsp almond butter**.

Snack total: 183 calories, 3 g protein, 24 g carbohydrate, 10 g fat, 1 g saturated fat, 0 mg cholesterol, 2 mg sodium, 4 g dietary fiber.

Lunch

Bean and Vegetable Soup with Salad (serves 4): In a large pot, cook according to package directions **¼ cup hulled barley, ¼ cup black-eyed peas**, and **¼ cup lentils,** in **vegetable broth.** During last 15 minutes of cooking, add **½ cup dried mushrooms, ½ cup chopped carrots, ½ cup chopped potato, ¼ tsp cumin,** and **2 to 3 crushed garlic cloves.** Garnish with **½ cup chopped scallions.** For a side salad, top **8 cups baby spinach** with **1 cup soy "bacon" bits, 1 cup shredded carrot,** and **4 Tbsp light Italian dressing.**

Lunch total per person: 324 calories, 32 g protein, 45 g carbohydrate, 3 g fat, 0 g saturated fat, 0 mg cholesterol, 1,395 mg sodium, 12 g dietary fiber.

Afternoon Snack

Add **a large sliced fresh peach** or **nectarine** to **1 cup low-fat plain yogurt** or **soy yogurt.** Top with **½ Tbsp wheat germ** and **1 Tbsp crystallized ginger.**

Snack total: 254 calories, 15 g protein, 41 g carbohydrate, 5 g fat, 2 g saturated fat, 14 mg cholesterol, 160 mg sodium, 3 g dietary fiber.

Dinner

Paprika Mashed Potatoes, and Vegetables with Cheese (serves 4): Gently boil **4 large unpeeled chopped red potatoes** for 15 minutes until done. Drain. Add **½ cup fat-free plain yogurt** (may use soy), **½ cup silken tofu, ½ Tbsp Hungarian paprika, ½ tsp freshly ground pepper,** and **salt** to taste. Mash or beat with an electric mixer until smooth. Top with **1 Tbsp olive oil** and **2 Tbsp parsley.** Serve with **4 cups steamed vegetables** such as broccoli, summer squash, and carrots, topped with **4 oz grated low-fat cheese** such as Mexican mix.

Dinner total per person: 336 calories, 18 g protein, 53 g carbohydrate, 8 g fat, 2 g saturated fat, 7 mg cholesterol, 104 mg sodium, 8 g dietary fiber.

....

Day 2 total: *1,438 calories, 89 g protein, 204 g carbohydrate, 37 g fat, 7 g saturated fat, 21 mg cholesterol, 2,327 mg sodium, 34 g dietary fiber.*

Day 3

Breakfast

Serve 2 waffles such as **Lifestream Hemp Plus Toaster Waffles** with **2 cups mixed fresh fruit** such as cantaloupe, kiwifruit, and blueberries.

Breakfast total: 326 calories, 7 g protein, 62 g carbohydrate, 7 g fat, 2 g saturated fat, 12 mg cholesterol, 584 mg sodium, 5 g dietary fiber.

Morning Snack

A **6-oz low-fat drinkable yogurt** (such as Dannon or Yoplait) or **soy yogurt** (such as Silk).

Snack total: 153 calories, 7 g protein, 27 g carbohydrate, 3 g fat, 2 g saturated fat, 9 mg cholesterol, 94 mg sodium, 0 g dietary fiber.

Lunch

Grilled Corn, Quinoa, and Spinach Salad (serves 4): Prepare **1½ cup quinoa** ahead of time. Cut corn from **2 ears fresh steamed** or **grilled corn** and toss with **1 15-oz can black beans**, drained, **½ cup roasted red peppers**, **½ cup low-fat feta cheese**, crumbled, **¼ cup minced red onion**, **½ cup walnut pieces**, **½ cucumber**, chopped, **¼ cup light salad dressing,** and **3 cups fresh baby spinach**.

Lunch total per person: 437 calories, 19 g protein, 59 g carbohydrate, 16 g fat, 3 g saturated fat, 10 mg cholesterol, 643 mg sodium, 12 g dietary fiber.

Afternoon Snack

A medium pear and **2 sticks low-fat string cheese** or **soy cheese**.

Snack total: 257 calories, 16 g protein, 27 g carbohydrate, 10 g fat, 6 g saturated fat, 31 mg cholesterol, 299 mg sodium, 4 g dietary fiber.

Dinner

Moroccan Spiced Stuffed Peppers with Vegetable Medley (serves 4): Prepare **1 cup cooked brown rice** ahead of time. Place **4 red or green bell peppers**, with tops removed and seeded, in a medium saucepan and cover with water. Simmer for 5 minutes. Remove from water and drain. Pour out water and reserve pan. Mix **1 package veggie burger** such as Boca Ground Burger, **½ cup organic vegetable broth, 6 to 8 preroasted and peeled jarred chestnuts**, thinly sliced, **2 tsp minced garlic, juice from ½ lemon, ¼ cup fresh mint**, finely chopped, **1 tsp ground cinnamon, ½ tsp ground cumin**, and **a few shakes Tabasco sauce**, and stuff into peppers. Pour an additional **½ cup vegetable broth** in pan and stand peppers in broth. Cover pan and simmer over low heat 15 to 20 minutes. Reserve broth for soup; it may be frozen. Use **fresh basil leaves** for garnish if desired. For a side dish, steam a **4-cup medley of vegetables** such as carrots, broccoli, and cauliflower. Top with **½ cup sesame seeds** and **2 Tbsp extra virgin olive oil**.

Dinner total per person: 424 calories, 24 g protein, 44 g carbohydrate, 19 g fat, 3 g saturated fat, 0 mg cholesterol, 576 mg sodium, 12 g dietary fiber.

....

Day 3 total: *1,597 calories, 73 g protein, 219 g carbohydrate, 55 g fat, 16 g saturated fat, 62 mg cholesterol, 2,196 mg sodium, 33 g dietary fiber.*

Day 4

Breakfast

Spread **1 Apple Cinnamon Bran Muffin** (see recipe below) with **1 Tbsp peanut** or **almond butter.** Serve with an **8-oz glass of orange-mango juice**.

Apple Cinnamon Bran Muffins (makes 12): Grate **2 large tart unpeeled apples** and toss with **1 tsp cinnamon.** Mix **2 cups bran flakes cereal, ½ cup texturized vegetable protein, ½ cup whole wheat flour, ¼ cup barley flour, ¼ cup brown rice flour**, and **1 cup fat-free milk** or **light soy milk** and allow to stand 5 minutes. Preheat oven to 350°F. Spray twelve 2½" muffin cups with **nonstick cooking spray.** In a large bowl, mix **2 Tbsp macadamia nut oil, 2 Tbsp flax meal, 1 Tbsp honey, ⅓ cup molasses, 1 tsp vanilla extract**, and cereal mixture. Fold in the apples and cinnamon. Fill the muffin pans and bake for 25 minutes. Muffins may be eaten fresh or frozen and reheated.

Breakfast total per person: 354 calories, 9 g protein, 56 g carbohydrate, 13 g fat, 2 g saturated fat, 0 mg cholesterol, 69 mg sodium, 5 g dietary fiber.

Morning Snack

A medium orange and **1 oz soy nuts.**

Snack total: 182 calories, 13 g protein, 24 g carbohydrate, 4 g fat, 1 g saturated fat, 0 mg cholesterol, 150 mg sodium, 8 g dietary fiber.

Lunch

Prepare a **veggie burger** (such as Morningstar Farms Mushroom Lovers patty or Spicy Black Bean burger) on **a 100% whole grain burger bun** (such as Sara Lee or Pepperidge Farm). Add **2 thick slices of tomatoes** (organic heirloom are best), **alfalfa sprouts, ¼ sliced avocado, ½ sliced cucumber**, and if desired, **2 tsp soy mayonnaise**. Serve with **1 cup mixed fresh fruit** such as kiwifruit, blackberries, oranges, and banana.

Lunch total (with mayonnaise): 487 calories, 19 g protein, 74 g carbohydrate, 17 g fat, 3 g saturated fat, 5 mg cholesterol, 718 mg sodium, 20 g dietary fiber.

Afternoon Snack

A 6-oz low-fat fruit yogurt or **soy yogurt** and **about 10 soy crisps.**

Snack total: 275 calories, 15 g protein, 47 g carbohydrate, 4 g fat, 1 g saturated fat, 7 mg cholesterol, 362 mg sodium, 2 g dietary fiber.

Dinner

Sliced "Chicken" with Ginger over Coconut Rice (serves 4): Cut 16 oz "chicken" seitan or Quorn "chicken" cutlets into thin strips. Peel and thinly slice **1 piece fresh ginger**, 4 to 5 inches long. Mix **1 Tbsp cornstarch** with **3 Tbsp water**. Coat a nonstick pan with **canola oil spray** and brown the seitan/cutlet strips. Add the ginger, **½ cup raw sliced mushrooms,** and ¾ cup water. Cook 5 minutes. Add the cornstarch, **1 Tbsp soy sauce**, and **1 Tbsp cognac**. Add **salt** and **pepper** to taste. Cook and stir until thickened. Serve with **4 cups mixed raw vegetables** such as cherry tomatoes, snow peas, and broccoli. For a side dish of coconut rice, prepare **2 cups cooked basmati brown rice** according to package directions, and substitute **light coconut milk** for half of the water.

Dinner total per person: 354 calories, 18 g protein, 35 g carbohydrate, 16 g fat, 7 g saturated fat, 2 mg cholesterol, 848 mg sodium, 7 g dietary fiber.

Day 4 total: *1,652 calories, 74 g protein, 236 g carbohydrate, 54 g fat, 14 g saturated fat, 14 mg cholesterol, 2,147 mg sodium, 42 g dietary fiber.*

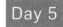

Day 5

⬊ *Breakfast*

Top ¾ **cup Back to Nature High Protein Crunch Cereal** with ½ **cup kefir and soy milk mix**. Add ½ **cup fresh organic berries** such as raspberries, strawberries, or blueberries. Serve with **8 oz pomegranate or cranberry juice**.

Breakfast total: 379 calories, 9 g protein, 90 g carbohydrate, 5 g fat, 0 g saturated fat, 0 mg cholesterol, 160 mg sodium, 14 g dietary fiber.

⬊ *Morning Snack*

2 oz low-fat Cheddar cheese or **soy cheese** and **4 or 5 whole wheat crackers.**

Snack total: 169 calories, 15 g protein, 12 g carbohydrate, 7 g fat, 3 g saturated fat, 12 mg cholesterol, 117 mg sodium, 2 g dietary fiber.

⬊ *Lunch*

Vegetarian Taco Salad (serves 4): Combine in a large bowl **4 cups torn romaine, Bibb, or spring mix lettuce, 1 cup chopped fresh tomatoes, 1 ripe avocado,** peeled and chopped, **1 cup diced tomatoes,** fresh or canned, and seasoned with **basil or cilantro, 2 scallions,** chopped, ⅔ **cup canned red kidney beans,** drained, ⅔ **cup shredded soy Cheddar cheese, ¼ cup sliced black olives**. For dressing, whisk together ⅓ **cup fresh salsa** and ⅓ **cup fat-free sour cream** or **soy yogurt**. Garnish with **1 oz** per person **reduced-fat tortilla chips** or **Trader Joe's Spicy Flax Soy Tortilla Chips.**

Lunch total per person: 366 calories, 17 g protein, 47 g carbohydrate, 14 g fat, 2 g saturated fat, 2 mg cholesterol, 953 mg sodium, 9 g dietary fiber.

Afternoon Snack

About 20 soy crisps and a medium nectarine.

Snack total: 269 calories, 15 g protein, 44 g carbohydrate, 5 g fat, 0 g saturated fat, 0 mg cholesterol, 527 mg sodium, 6 g dietary fiber.

Dinner

Mexican Brown Rice (serves 4): Saute **1 cup uncooked brown rice** and ¾ **cup finely chopped yellow onion** in **1 Tbsp olive oil** in a medium nonstick pan for 3 minutes. Stir in **1½ cups organic vegetable broth, 1 tsp minced garlic, 2 tsp chili powder, 1½ cups diced tomatoes,** fresh or canned, **1 finely chopped bell pepper of any color, salt,** and **pepper** to taste, and cook about 45 minutes until rice is soft.

Red Beans (serves 4): Rinse ½ **lb dry red beans** and add to **4 cups water** with **2 bay leaves**. Cook until tender, about 1½ hours. Add **1 large chopped onion, 4 ribs chopped celery, 1 chopped green pepper, ½ tsp garlic powder, ½ tsp oregano, ½ tsp thyme, ½ tsp cumin, salt, and pepper** to taste, and cook over low heat for 15 minutes. Stir in ⅓ **cup finely chopped parsley** and cook for 1 minute. Remove bay leaves before serving.

Dinner total per person: 448 calories, 17 g protein, 86 g carbohydrate, 6 g fat, 0 g saturated fat, 0 mg cholesterol, 222 mg sodium, 13 g dietary fiber.

···

Day 5 total: *1,631 calories, 73 g protein, 279 g carbohydrate, 37 g fat, 5 g saturated fat, 14 mg cholesterol, 1,979 mg sodium, 44 g dietary fiber.*

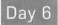

Day 6

Breakfast

Health Smoothie (serves 1): Blend until smooth ½ **banana, 6 to 8 strawberries, 1 scoop protein powder, ¼ cup oat bran, 1 Tbsp flax meal, 1 Tbsp powdered greens** (such as sprouted barley, wheat grass, chlorella, or kelp), or grains and ½ **cup soy milk** or **organic cow's milk.**

Breakfast total: 378 calories, 31 g protein, 56 g carbohydrate, 9 g fat, 2 g saturated fat, 0 mg cholesterol, 319 mg sodium, 11 g dietary fiber.

Morning Snack

2 oz low-fat Cheddar cheese or **soy cheese.**

Snack total: 98 calories, 14 g protein, 1 g carbohydrate, 4 g fat, 3 g saturated fat, 12 mg cholesterol, 352 mg sodium, 0 g dietary fiber.

Lunch

Carrot Soufflé (serves 4): Cook **1 lb carrots** until very tender. Place in food processor and process until smooth. Add **3 Tbsp evaporated cane juice, 2 Tbsp fat-free sour cream, 1½ Tbsp flour, 1 Tbsp olive oil, ½ tsp baking powder, ½ tsp vanilla extract, ⅛ tsp salt,** and **2 medium eggs** and pulse to combine. Spoon mixture into a 1 qt soufflé dish coated with **nonstick cooking spray**. Bake at 350°F for about 30 minutes or until puffed and set.

Grilled Cheese Sandwiches (serves 4): For each of 4 sandwiches, place **2 low-fat or fat-free cheese slices** (American, Swiss, or Monterey Jack) between **2 slices whole grain bread**. Spray a nonstick griddle with **olive oil** and lightly grill the sandwiches, turning to brown both sides. When cheese has melted, remove from pan and open the sandwiches to fill with **thick tomato slices, alfalfa sprouts, or sandwich pickles**.

Lunch total per person: 436 calories, 25 g protein, 57 g carbohydrate, 13 g fat, 5 g saturated fat, 119 mg cholesterol, 771 mg sodium, 8 g dietary fiber.

Afternoon Snack

A ¼-cup mix of raisins and peanuts (half-and-half mix).

Snack total: 180 calories, 5 g protein, 17 g carbohydrate, 10 g fat, 3 g saturated fat, 0 mg cholesterol, 117 mg sodium, 2 g dietary fiber.

Dinner

Vegetable Risotto (serves 4): Coat a small baking dish with **olive oil cooking spray**. In a large saucepan, cook **1 small chopped onion** in **1 Tbsp olive oil** for 2 minutes. Add **½ cup Arborio rice** and cook 2 minutes longer. Add **1 cup organic vegetable broth** and bring to boil for 3 minutes. Stir in **1 cup sliced portobello mushrooms, 1 cup chopped asparagus, ¼ cup dried cranberries, 1 Tbsp fresh**

minced basil leaves, and **2 Tbsp finely grated Parmesan cheese** or **soy cheese**. Cover and bake for 30 minutes at 425°F.

Sweet Potato Pancakes (serves 4): Mix **3 cups peeled and finely shredded sweet potatoes** or **yams,** ½ **cup finely chopped onion,** ¾ **cup whole wheat pastry flour,** ½ **tsp no-salt herb blend,** ¼ **cup chopped parsley, 1 cup finely shredded zucchini, juice of** ½ **lemon,** and ¾ **cup egg substitute.** In a large nonstick skillet, warm **2 tsp olive** or **canola oil** over medium heat. Drop large spoonfuls of the batter onto the pan to form thin pancakes. Cook each side about 2 minutes or until golden brown and crispy. Keep cooked pancakes warm in a warm oven until all the batter has been used. Serve with **1 cup unsweetened applesauce per person**.

Dinner total per person: 569 calories, 17 g protein, 106 g carbohydrate, 9 g fat, 2 g saturated fat, 3 mg cholesterol, 269 mg sodium, 13 g dietary fiber.

Day 6 total: *1,661 calories, 92 g protein, 237 g carbohydrate, 45 g fat, 15 g saturated fat, 134 mg cholesterol, 1,828 mg sodium, 34 g dietary fiber.*

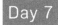

Day 7

⇘ *Breakfast*

Pineapple Cheesecake (serves 4): Preheat oven to 350°F. Layer **1 cup bread cubes** in a 1-qt casserole dish. In a small saucepan, combine **juice from 1 cup crushed drained pineapple** with **2 tsp cornstarch**. Heat and stir until the mixture becomes clear. Set aside. In a medium bowl, stir together **1 cup part-skim ricotta cheese, 1 Tbsp flax meal**, and **1 cup crushed drained pineapple**. Add the cornstarch mixture. Spoon on top of the bread cubes. Combine **1 Tbsp wheat germ, 2 Tbsp dried bread crumbs,** and **2 Tbsp brown sugar** and sprinkle over the cheesecake batter. Bake 30 to 35 minutes.

Breakfast total per person: 224 calories, 10 g protein, 33 g carbohydrate, 7 g fat, 4 g saturated fat, 19 mg cholesterol, 198 mg sodium, 3 g dietary fiber.

Morning Snack

A bowl of **mixed fresh fruit: a sliced banana, a sliced nectarine, and 1 cup blueberries.**

Snack total: 256 calories, 3 g protein, 64 g carbohydrate, 2 g fat, 0 g saturated fat, 0 mg cholesterol, 10 mg sodium, 9 g dietary fiber.

Lunch

Curried Potatoes, Cauliflower, and Peas (serves 4): Cook **1 chili pepper, 1 Tbsp grated fresh ginger, 1 tsp crushed garlic,** and **1 small chopped onion** in **2 Tbsp olive oil** for 2 minutes. Add **1 lb unpeeled red potatoes**, cut into ¼" slices to make about 2½ cups, and cook 10 minutes longer, stirring. Add **3 cups cauliflower pieces** and cook 5 minutes longer. Add **2 small boxes thawed frozen peas, 1 tsp curry powder, ½ tsp ground cumin, 2 Tbsp chopped fresh cilantro, juice of 1 lime,** and **½ cup vegetarian soup stock**. Cover and cook until potatoes are done, about 5 to 10 minutes.

Lunch total per person: 273 calories, 11 g protein, 41 g carbohydrate, 8 g fat, 1 g saturated fat, 0 mg cholesterol, 480 mg sodium, 13 g dietary fiber.

Afternoon Snack

6 or 7 Wasa crackers with **1 Tbsp peanut butter.**

Snack total: 262 calories, 9 g protein, 34 g carbohydrate, 11 g fat, 2 g saturated fat, 0 mg cholesterol, 342 mg sodium, 4 g dietary fiber.

Dinner

Mandarin Salad with Tempeh (serves 4): Prepare ahead. For the marinade, combine in a shallow pan **2 Tbsp orange marmalade, 1 tsp minced fresh ginger, 1 tsp minced garlic, juice of ½ lemon and ½ lime, ⅓ cup orange juice, ¼ cup soy sauce,** and **¼ tsp ground red pepper**. Cut **1 lb tempeh** into 2" by ½" strips and microwave for 5 minutes. Cover with marinade and refrigerate for at least 2 hours or overnight. Turn tempeh to coat evenly.

In a large salad bowl, toss **4 cups mixed salad greens**, **1 coarsely grated carrot**, **6 sliced radishes**, **1 small jar artichoke hearts**, and **1 cup mandarin orange segments**. Remove tempeh with a slotted spoon and add to salad ingredients. Mix ½ **cup fat-free plain yogurt** into marinade to form a dressing, then drizzle over salad.

Dinner total per person: 336 calories, 27 g protein, 36 g carbohydrate, 13 g fat, 3 g saturated fat, 0 mg cholesterol, 1,400 mg sodium, 12 g dietary fiber.

....

<u>Day 7 total:</u> *1,351 calories, 60 g protein, 208 g carbohydrate, 41 g fat, 10 g saturated fat, 19 mg cholesterol, 2,430 mg sodium, 41 g dietary fiber.*

SHOPPING LIST FOR MENUS FOR VEGETARIANS

- **Vegetables**: 10 to 12 potatoes or yams, red potatoes, 4 to 6 tomatoes, 1 box cherry tomatoes, 8 to 10 red or green bell peppers, 1 or 2 bags carrots, several containers fresh baby spinach, 1 bunch fresh parsley, several large onions and scallions, 1 bunch broccoli,1 cauliflower, sugar snap peas, 1 eggplant, 1 acorn squash, 1 summer squash, 1 box raw mushrooms, portobello mushrooms, 1 container dried mushrooms, 2 zucchini, 2 to 4 ears fresh corn, 2 or 3 cucumbers, small container sprouts, 2 avocados, 1 head romaine lettuce, several ribs celery, asparagus, 6 radishes, 1 chili pepper, 2 packages frozen peas, 1 jar artichoke hearts, snow peas, 1 package mixed salad greens.
- **Fruit**: Several bananas, apples, cantaloupe, oranges, lemons, limes, pears, peaches, nectarines, and kiwifruits, 1 pineapple, several boxes berries (such as blueberries, strawberries, raspberries, or blackberries), several boxes dried fruit (such as raisins, cherries, cranberries, blueberries, figs, prunes, or apricots), 1 jar unsweetened applesauce, 1 can mandarin orange segments.
- **Juice**: Several containers of juice such as orange, pomegranate, orange-mango, or cranberry juice.
- **Legumes**: 2 15-oz cans black beans, 1 15-oz can chickpeas, 1 15-oz can red kidney beans, dried black-eyed peas, dried lentils, dried red beans, peanuts.
- **Whole grains**: 1 box high-protein oatmeal, 1 box oat bran, 1 loaf whole grain bread, 1 pack whole grain pita bread, several whole grain bagels, 1 pack whole grain waffles, 1 pack whole grain buns, 1 box whole wheat crackers, 1 box brown rice, 1 box Arborio rice,

1 box rotini pasta, 1 box bulgur, 1 box hulled barley, 1 container quinoa, 1 box bran flakes cereal, 1 box Back to Nature High Protein Crunch Cereal, 1 box Wasa crackers.

- **Meat alternatives:** 2 lb veggie burger such as Boca Ground Burger, 1 lb "chicken" seitan or Quorn "chicken" cutlets, 1 lb tempeh, 3 oz soy sausage patty, 1 jar soy "bacon" bits.
- **Dairy and soy products**: 1 container kefir, ½ gal soy milk, or fat-free or low-fat cow's milk, several large containers fat-free or low-fat plain yogurt, 1 container tofu, 16 oz low-fat or fat-free cheese, several 6-oz low-fat fruit yogurts or soy yogurts, several drinkable yogurts, 8 oz low-fat feta cheese, 1 container low-fat or fat-free sour cream, 8 oz Parmesan cheese, 8 oz low-fat cottage or ricotta cheese, string cheese, 1 package shredded soy Cheddar cheese.
- **Eggs**: 1 dozen eggs, 1 16-oz container Egg Beaters.
- **Oils**: Olive oil, macadamia nut oil, canola or olive oil cooking spray.
- **Nuts and seeds**: Walnuts, 1 jar chestnuts, sesame seeds, soy nuts, 1 jar almond or peanut butter, 1 jar tahini.
- **Spices**: Garlic powder, fresh garlic, fresh basil, dried herb seasoning such as Mrs. Dash, salt, pepper, crystallized ginger, fresh ginger, paprika, fresh mint, ground cumin, cinnamon, chili powder, oregano, thyme, cilantro, curry powder, ground red pepper, Tabasco sauce, soy sauce, vanilla extract, bay leaves.
- **Baking ingredients**: Wheat germ, texturized vegetable protein, whole wheat flour, barley flour, brown rice flour, wheat bran, flax meal, honey, molasses, evaporated cane juice, brown sugar, cornstarch, cognac, 1 pint light coconut milk, protein powder, powdered greens, baking powder, bread crumbs, several cans organic vegetable broth.
- **Other**: 2 bags baked tortilla chips or soy crisps, plant sterol spread, light Italian salad dressing, soy mayonnaise, small container black olives, 1 salsa, 1 jar orange marmalade.

DOCUMENT LOCATOR

LOCATION OF IMPORTANT DOCUMENTS

FOR _____

Social Security No._____–_____–_____

Spouse _____

Social Security No._____–_____–_____

My valuable papers and assets are stored in these locations:

(A) Residence (Where) _____

(B) Safe Deposit Box _____

(Bank) (Address)

(C) Lawyer's Office _____

(Address)

(D) _____

(E) _____

Note: Place location letter in (   ) below.

ITEM LOCATION	ITEM LOCATION	ITEM LOCATION
Will (original) ( )	Umbrella policy ( )	Auto ownership records ( )
Will (copy) ( )	Disability insurance ( )	Mortgage agreement ( )
Trust agreements ( )	Employment contracts ( )	Real estate titles and deeds ( )
Power of Attorney (POA) ( )	Partnership agreements ( )	Title insurance ( )
Medical directive ( )	Business records ( )	Mortgage agreement ( )
Burial instructions ( )	Net worth statement ( )	Rental property records ( )
Cemetery plot deed ( )	Tax returns ( )	Loan agreements ( )
Spouse's will (original) ( )	Bank statements ( )	Home contents list ( )
Spouse's will (copy) ( )	Credit card list ( )	Boat ownership records ( )
Spouse's POA ( )	Certificates of Deposit ( )	Warranty records ( )
Spouse's medical directive ( )	Checkbook ( )	Birth certificates ( )
Spouse's burial instructions ( )	Savings passbook ( )	Adoption papers ( )
Children's guardian document ( )	Record of investments ( )	Diplomas ( )
Letter of instruction ( )	Stock certificates ( )	Discharge papers ( )
Safe combination ( )	Mutual funds ( )	Marriage certificate ( )
Safety deposit box ( )	Bonds ( )	Separation records ( )
Social Security card ( )	Other securities ( )	Divorce records ( )
Life insurance, group ( )	Retirement plans ( )	Citizenship papers ( )
Life insurance, individual ( )	Annuity contracts ( )	List of relatives and friends ( )
Other death benefits ( )	Stock option plans ( )	List of advisors ( )
Health insurance policy ( )	Stock purchase plan ( )	Professional memberships ( )
Auto insurance policy ( )	Profit sharing plan ( )	Medical records ( )
Homeowners policy ( )	Savings bonds ( )	Computer passwords ( )
Long-term care insurance policy ( )		( ) PIN numbers ( )

HARVARD FINANCIAL EDUCATORS, PO BOX 304, HARVARD, MA 01451 / www.deelee.net

ACKNOWLEDGMENTS

Writing this book was quite an adventure. I recall with a smile on my face when I actually conceptualized the theme and title while walking around a reservoir with my sidekick Mary Jane Ryan, my kindred spirit and writing companion. I am double blessed with MJ in my life, both as a colleague and a friend. The Rodale team was headed by my formidable captain Mariska van Aalst, editor par excellence, as well as the keeper of the clock. Kudos to Mariska for another terrific job well done. Of course, nothing would be possible without my wondrous literary agent Amanda Urban calling the shots from ICM. This book was truly a collaborative effort. I am deeply grateful to Carla Sottovia, PhD, and Ken Cooper, MD, of the Cooper Institute for their terrific leadership compiling the exercise data. Words of wisdom were truly appreciated from Elaine Cress, PhD, and Robert Schwartz, MD, both pioneers in the field of geriatrics and physical activity. Elizabeth Pradhan, PhD, and Amy Anderson provided critical epidemiologic data while the financial whiz kids included Prudential's Maria Umbach and Mary Flowers. I am so thankful for ongoing feedback and advice from my army of brilliant minds and great friends, including Jim Hill, PhD; Mehmet Oz, MD; Dean Ornish, MD; Ken Cooper, MD; Andrew Weil, MD; George Chrousos, MD; and Christiane Northrup, MD. My Peeke Performance team was superb in keeping me on track and patiently supporting me. Torne Jacobson and Loren Creamer were my stabilizing spirits who succeeded in maintaining my sanity when my daily schedule looked like a mission impossible. Finally, no one knows better what it took to make this book happen than my amazing family. Aunt Eva, Eliot Pearl, and Eric Echenrode always had an endless supply of affirmations and encouragement. Greg and Emma kept me rooted in what is important in life. Linda Solheim; Kay Kirkpatrick, MD; Art and Sheila and Naomi Henderson were the sanity squad I have always relied upon. And throughout it all, my husband, Mark, endured the marathon writing sessions and canceled vacations, keeping me centered and loved. As I write this, I realize how blessed I truly am.

INDEX

Underscored page references indicate boxed text and tables.
Boldface references indicate photographs.

WITHDRAWN